Party**Walls**
A practical guide

RIBA ∰ **Publishing**

Nicol Stuart Morrow Dip Arch ARIBA

Published by RIBA Publishing, 15 Bonhill Street,
London EC2P 2EA

This edition is an expanded and updated edition of
The Party Walls Workbook, first published in 1998.

ISBN 978 1 85946 310 9

Stock Code 69967

British Library Cataloguing-in-Publication Data
A catalogue record for this book is available
from the British Library.

Publisher: Steven Cross
Commissioning Editor: James Thompson
Project Editor: Anna Walters
Editor: Paul Beverley
Designed by Kneath Associates
Typeset by Academic + Technical, Bristol
Printed and bound by Polestar Wheaton's, Exeter

RIBA Publishing is part of RIBA Enterprises Ltd.

www.ribaenterprises.com

The masculine pronoun 'he' is used throughout
this text, rather than the neutral term 'he/she'.
This is in order to follow the convention used in
the Party Wall etc. Act 1996 itself, and it should
be inferred that the author refers to any individual
person regardless of gender.

Preface

Since the middle of the nineteenth century disputes involving construction work relating to property situated in the Inner London Boroughs, particularly those involving party walls, floors or excavations affecting adjoining or adjacent property, had been resolved under the control of successive statutes legislated by Parliament, the final one being the London Building Acts (Amendment) Act 1939.

Before 1996, resolving problems arising from work concerned with party walls in areas remote from the London Boroughs having District Surveyors' jurisdiction often depended on applying common law to largely technical matters; implementing the procedures involved, of necessity, the costly engagement of the legal profession to an extent often sufficient to materially and adversely affect the finances of the parties involved.

The Party Wall etc. Act 1996 extends the application of the statute to the whole of England and Wales and it is evident to observant construction professionals, especially architects practising in these regions, that not to acquire at least a working knowledge of the legislation must be considered not only dilatory but, in its omission, might also deprive a client of the duty of care to which he is entitled.

The resolution of the many and varied technical and legal problems involving party structures, adjacent structures and boundaries have hitherto not often been found to have been foremost in the architect's mind and are more likely to have been thought of as matters to be later dealt with by specialist surveyors or lawyers. This book aims to correct this misconception. Acquiring knowledge of the details of ownership of properties, their legal titles and the limits of their environs is a requirement essential for the architect to identify the priorities governing his project and to establish information which will influence the design.

A client gains little benefit to learn, too late, that consequent on inadequate discovery of adjoining interests the design he has approved has been compromised, might require expensive modifications and in some circumstances might be unviable. In cities, especially, it is sometimes unavoidable that a development has to be placed adjacent to a building in multi-occupation where the many adjoining owners may all be entitled to separately receive notice of the building owner's intentions; the architect, well positioned in the design process to make reasonable assessment of the costs involved in complying with the Act, will perhaps modify or adjust the design so as to make it conform and also offer the client the advice necessary to balance the commercial options of compliance or avoidance.

The architect should be competent in explaining to his client the practical applications of the Act and why its mandatory procedures would seem to conflict with the dictums relating to property and rights of possession, the entrenched right to deny access to property and at the same time oblige him to not oppose the actions he always has understood to constitute trespass.

It would be fair to say that, having received a building owner's statutory notices, owners are unlikely to remain unbiased or be willing to allow work to proceed on their property without wishing to be personally involved; it is for these reasons that they are not permitted to act on their own behalf but have to stand aside and are obliged to appoint surveyors who, while acting for them, must remain neutral and proceed only in accordance with the provisions of the Act.

Acknowledgements

In writing this book, and particularly in writing those chapters concerning the quasi-legal status of the appointed party wall surveyor it has been necessary that I seek legal opinion on these matters. In this regard I have to sincerely thank Jonathan Steinert of Counsel for his erudite advice which has been instrumental when, in considering the role of the surveyor in relation to the law, I take a different view from that held by others in the legal profession.

I also thank my friends, the members of the Pyramus & Thisbe Club with whom I enjoy many debates, usually on some of the more equivocal aspects of the Act, and especially I thank Andrew Smith, Solicitor, who answers my calls for advice and never seems to mind me interrupting his busy day.

Contents

Overview of the Act

Overview of the Act

The Party Wall etc. Act came into force on 1 July 1997 and, with the exception of Inns of Court properties in London, it extends to the whole of England and Wales. Part V1 of the London Building Acts (Amendment) Act 1939 and relevant sections of the Bristol Improvement Act 1847 (and as later amended) are repealed.

The Act sets out the rights and obligations of property owners involved in the building of party structures or their repair and alteration, and also those concerned with excavation carried out within notifiable distances from buildings on adjoining land. The Act sets out the procedures for notification of proposed work and protocols for the obligatory appointment of surveyors when disputes need to be resolved.

New building on line of junction (Section 1)

- Notice of at least one month must be served on an adjoining owner before building a new wall on the line of junction.

- If agreed by the adjoining owner, the wall may be built astride the boundary line and it is then either a party wall or a party fence wall.

- The costs for the work involved are to be shared between the parties in agreed proportions and, in the event that agreement cannot be reached, surveyors must be appointed under the provisions of Section 10 to resolve the matters by award.

- If the adjoining owner does not consent to the wall being a party wall the building owner must not build it astride the boundary but, at his own cost, entirely on his own land, and be entirely responsible for compensating any adjoining owners or occupiers for any damage caused by his works.

- In this section, dissent by the adjoining owner does not constitute a dispute under the meaning of the Act, so there is no obligation to appoint surveyors, but as the right is given to place footings and foundations over the boundary and under the adjoining owner's land within 12 months from service of notice, the extent or construction of the foundations might be disputed, and this in itself would lead to the appointment of surveyors.

Repairs etc. of party wall: rights of owner (Section 2)

- A building owner has the right to underpin, demolish, repair, raise, lower or rebuild a party wall when such works are necessitated by its poor condition or because of his need for a higher or stronger wall.

- The right could also include for the cutting of chases or pockets into a wall for joist seatings or for the insertion of damp-proof courses, flashings or weatherings or for the cutting away of projections overhanging the building owner's land.

- Chimney stacks or flues belonging to the adjoining owner and being integral with the party structure must be maintained in working condition if the adjoining owner so requires.

- The right is given to expose a party wall or party structure hitherto enclosed, but accordingly it must be adequately protected either on a temporary basis or permanently if no enclosing work is built or intended to be built against it.

- The right is exercisable provided that proper written notice is given to all adjoining owners, all necessary protection is provided to the adjoining property, all safety legislation is complied with and any resultant damage is made good. There is provision for the adjoining owner to opt for compensation to be paid in lieu of having the damage made good.

Party structure notices (Section 3)

- Before a building owner may exercise any right given to him in Section 2 and, unless he has written consent from the adjoining owner to carry out work to the structure or needs to comply with a statutory notice relating to it being in a neglected or dangerous condition, he must serve on the adjoining owner a 'party structure notice'.

- The notice must state the building owner's name and address, give a description of the proposed works, its proposed starting date and, if the works include proposals to construct special foundations, be accompanied by drawings and details of the special foundations and include details of the loads they are to carry.

- The notice must be served at least two months before the commencement date of the work, and it will expire if the work is not started and proceeded with diligently within the 12 months following the date of its service.

Counter notices (Section 4)

- On receipt of a party structure notice served under Section 3, an adjoining owner may wish to serve a counter notice which proposes extra work to be carried out for his own benefit or perhaps, if he has given consent for their construction, to require modifications to the building owner's proposed special foundations.

- The counter notice giving the specification of the required work together with relevant drawings and details must be served by the adjoining owner within one month from the date of his receipt of the party structure notice. Unless compliance with the requested work would be injurious to the building owner, cause him unnecessary inconvenience or would unnecessarily delay his proposed works, he must comply with the terms of the counter notice.

Disputes arising under Section 3 and 4 (sSection 5)

- Any dispute, or deemed dispute, arising between the owners in respect of work to party walls must be resolved via the statutory appointment of a surveyor or surveyors under the provisions of Section 10.

Adjacent excavation and construction (Section 6)

- If a building owner's proposed works involve either temporary or permanent excavation and construction within 3 metres or 6 metres of an adjoining owner's building or structure, and at depths lower than their foundations, the building owner must serve notice of the proposals.

- The building owner may at his own expense or consequent to a request by the adjoining owner, underpin or otherwise strengthen or safeguard the foundations of the adjoining owner's building or structure.

- Where there exists more than one building or structure within the respective 3- and 6-metre horizontally measured distances from the building owner's proposed works, the properties might be in different ownerships and in these circumstances all relevant owners are deemed to be adjoining owners and each is entitled to receive written notice of the proposals.

- The building owner must serve notice on all or any adjoining owners, and must state whether he intends to underpin or otherwise strengthen or safeguard the foundations of the relevant adjoining buildings or structures. The notice, together with drawings showing the site and depth of the excavations and, if the intention is to erect a building or structure, its site, must be served at least one month before beginning the excavations.

- The notice will expire 12 months from the date of its service and therefore excavations must be started within that year and, on its completion and if so requested, the building owner shall supply to the adjoining owner drawings and particulars of the work as executed.

- The building owner is entirely liable to any adjoining owner or occupier for any injury they have suffered and which was caused by his work.

Compensation etc. (Section 7)

- A building owner is not entitled to cause unnecessary inconvenience to any adjoining owner or occupier.

- Where the building owner's work results in loss or damage to any adjoining owner or adjoining occupier he shall accordingly compensate them.

- Where the building owner lays open any part of an adjoining owner's land or buildings he must at his own expense provide adequate and necessary hoardings and shoring, and take any other measures to ensure the protection of the adjoining land or buildings and the security of any adjoining occupier.

- Without obtaining prior written consent the building owner is not entitled to place special foundations on an adjoining owner's land.

- Any work authorised by the Act must comply with statutory requirements and be carried out entirely in accordance with the drawn details agreed between the owners or, in the event of a dispute, by surveyors appointed on their behalf (Section 10).

Rights of entry (Section 8)

- Having first served notice a building owner, his workmen, agents and party wall surveyor are given the right to enter on any land or premises and to remain there for as long as is necessary to carry out any work authorised by the Act; any other action may be taken for that purpose including the removal of furniture and fittings.

- In emergency, and should access be unavailable, notice of the intention to enter must be given as soon as is practical and, accompanied by a police officer, forced entry may be effected. In other circumstances, perhaps to carry out works specified in a counter notice, the required period of notice to enter is 14 days.

Easements (Section 9)

- Easements such as rights to light, air or to support are not affected by work authorised by the Act and, further to the demolition of a party wall, will allow the continuation of the right to be incorporated in the rebuilt party wall.

- The right to maintain overhanging eaves or projecting foundations can be extinguished if the provisions of Section 2(2)(g) are invoked.

Resolution of disputes (Section 10)

- Serving notice in compliance with the Act often gives rise to disputes between owners, and these must be resolved by the appointment of surveyors.

- The first option is to appoint one surveyor, the "agreed surveyor" who will act impartially for both parties equally.

- The more usual option is for the parties to each individually appoint a surveyor and the two appointed surveyors will then select a third surveyor, a form of umpire, to determine matters when they cannot agree between themselves.

- All appointments must be made in writing and shall not be rescinded by either of the parties.

- If either party refuses or neglects to appoint a surveyor within 10 days of being so requested, then the other party is entitled to make the appointment on their behalf.

- If an agreed surveyor dies, refuses to act or fails to act within 10 days of being so requested then proceedings must start afresh.

- If an appointed surveyor dies or becomes incapable of acting then the party who appointed him may appoint a replacement. If an appointed surveyor refuses to act effectively within 10 days of a request so to do then the other surveyor may act *ex parte* to determine on the subject matter of the dispute.

- Where a third surveyor refuses or is unable to act then another shall forthwith be selected by the appointed surveyors.

- Where an appointed surveyor refuses to select a third surveyor the selection can be referred to the 'appointing officer' of the local authority.

- The appointed surveyors are charged with settling only the matters in dispute and which relate to work authorised by the Act.

- Decisions are set out in a party wall award and may include such matters as:

  - the right under the Act to carry out specific work
  - conditions relating to timing and manner of carrying out work
  - other related matters concerned with surveyors' fees and expenses incurred in making the award

- The award must be served forthwith on the parties by the surveyors or, should he be involved in the matter and after having received his fee, by the third surveyor.

- The award is conclusive but, within 14 days of its receipt, the parties have the right to appeal it to the county court. The court has powers to rescind it or modify it and may make such orders as to costs as it thinks fit.

Expenses and account for work carried out (Sections 11 and 13)

- Other than when the parties have agreed to share costs, say, of building or repairing a party wall, the general rule is that the building owner who wishes to carry out the work will pay them.

- When costs are shared, the determining factors in deciding the proportion for which each party might be liable could include their responsibility for the repair of defects or perhaps for the benefit they derive from the use made of the work.

- Other contributions could be payable to an adjoining owner as a fair allowance for disturbance or inconvenience caused by the work or the effect it has on his property or his business, and when he opts to take payment in lieu of having repairs made to damage caused by the building owner's work; he may also be required to make a contribution when he has to pay the costs incurred by the building owner who complies with the requirements of a counter notice or a request to underpin his building (Section 6).

- An adjoining owner may also be required to make a proportional payment to the building owner when he makes use of a party wall built and paid for solely by the building owner.

- An adjoining owner is entitled to be reimbursed the additional costs he sustains in carrying out his own development and where extra work is directly attributable to the special foundations placed on his land by the building owner.

- Contributions due from the adjoining owner are the subject of accounts submitted by the building owner within two months from completion of the related work, and if the adjoining owner raises no objection to the accounts within one month of their receipt they become payable.

- Should there be a failure to pay the due sum it would be recoverable through normal court procedures and until the due accounts are paid the property in any works carried out will remain solely with the building owner.

- If there is failure to pay an awarded sum, and the award has not been appealed to the county court, the sum is recoverable through the procedures of the magistrates' court.

- Disputes arising over responsibility for costs, expenses and matters to do with liability or apportionment between the parties are to be determined by the party wall surveyors in accordance with Section 10.

Security for expenses (Section 12)

- In the event that a property might change hands during the course of the works, or that the possibility arises of either owner's financial stability being doubted, the Act provides for an appropriate sum to be deposited as security for expenses against default by either of the owners.

- A situation might arise where an adjoining owner could be left in a difficult situation should the building owner be unable to fully discharge his obligations or, conversely, a building owner might be uncertain of the adjoining owner's ability to contribute to the cost of additional work he required under a counter notice.

- In all cases where a party has a requirement for security for expenses, notice must be served on the other party prior to and in advance of commencement of any work to which the security relates.

- Should a dispute arise as to justification of the proposed security or its amount or for any other related matter on which the parties cannot agree between themselves, it must be resolved by party wall surveyors under the provisions of Section 10.

Architects and the Party Wall etc. Act 1996

Architects and the Party Wall etc. Act 1996

Ever increasing legislation that governs and controls the work of most professionals has resulted in the architect – traditionally the designer of the project, coordinating his work with that of other professionals – now having also to be concerned with areas of expertise historically the preserve of other specialists and consultants, building surveyors, party wall surveyors and solicitors.

Other than for certain types of appointment – for example, those under design/ build contracts where their responsibilities are circumscribed – practising architects are required to maintain a working knowledge of relevant applicable legislation that could affect the work on which they are engaged. In particular, because compliance with the requirements of the Party Wall etc. Act 1996 is to be so frequently a part of the design of projects in urban areas, it may now be appropriate to include a general appreciation of the provisions and constraints of the Act as a core curriculum subject of compulsory professional development.

Ignorance of the procedures laid down by the Act could result in serious consequences both for the architect and for the client.

The influence of the Act on building design

Because of their ability to influence and control almost all critical aspects of their work from the beginning of its design stages, architects are generally better placed than other consultants, perhaps as party wall surveyors, to advise their clients on adjoining interests and on matters that will dictate the form a project will take. They are in a position to progress and modify preliminary designs so as to avoid unnecessary controversy and to lessen or even avoid a considerable proportion of the costs that are incurred when having to comply with the legislation.

If matters to be decided concern a party wall or other parts of premises shared with a neighbour, there is very little scope under Section 2 to do anything other than to comply with the Act's provisions although, for example under Section 6, there might be the opportunity to adjust the design so as to take it outside the Act's remit altogether.

Notice must be given if, say, it is proposed to excavate adjacent to an adjoining owner's premises for the purpose of constructing foundations and ground beams just within the prescribed horizontal distances defined in Section 6 and at a level deeper than the bottom of the foundations of the adjoining owner's building.

At an early stage, an architect should be able to assess the consequences of implementing a design that might be adversely affected by adjoining interests and one which will involve the client in considerable expenditure when the elements of its construction make service of notice obligatory; it makes common sense to ask the structural engineer to add some steel reinforcement to the ground beams, offset them to put them outside the prescribed distance and therefore obviate the need to serve a three-metre notice.

Architects and the Party Wall etc. Act 1996

11

The architect is best placed to decide the format of the design and has a considerable advantage over consultants who are appointed later, and perhaps as party wall surveyors, through being able to mitigate the potentially expensive effect of the client's work on the adjoining owner's property.

The architect's role as party wall surveyor

For architects acting as party wall surveyors there are some interesting shifts in roles and relationships to be noted.

Architects who advise clients about adjoining interests, ownerships, leases, title, service of notices, boundaries and the effect of the client's proposals on adjoining land etc. will be expected to offer no less professionalism and duty of care than they are required to provide in everyday architectural practice.

Professional indemnity insurers will need to be satisfied that the architect is competent to undertake this specialised work, and architects will need confirmation that appropriate PII cover can be obtained.

When the adjoining owner's dissent to a notice leads to the mandatory appointment of surveyors, and the architect is appointed by the client to act as his party wall surveyor, then other than in very limited situations the client himself is not permitted to be involved in the resolution of the disputed matters.

The appointed surveyor's duty is to carry out the provisions of the Act, act impartially between the parties in dispute, and settle matters by award. The provisions of the award may be appealed by the owners, and this possibility in itself tends to reduce the risk of any liability in negligence attaching to an architect appointed as a party wall surveyor, especially since the appointment is to fulfil a statutory function and is not an appointment to represent a client.

Avoiding conflicts of interest

It is easy to understand the apparent contradictions in circumstances when the building owner, the originator of the served notice, having received no written consent to his proposals has to accept that his architect/agent, probably the person who drafted the notice in the first place, has now become his appointed surveyor.

The change of role from architect/agent to appointed surveyor is significant.

The architect having acted entirely on his client's behalf, up to and including the mandatory service of notice, is now, as a party wall surveyor, being required to act impartially between the owners. In addition, he has a statutory duty to consider the welfare of the adjoining owner, the adjoining owner's property and certainly his everyday environment, all of which are soon to be substantially affected by the building owner's works.

How then might then an architect/surveyor maintain this perhaps contradictory position while also having to consider accepting an appointment to act impartially when, as an example:

(a) The owner might be a client of substance whose business involves the architect's day-to-day work and whose development projects are carried out by the architects firm; or

(b) The architect is engaged on behalf of a client on a building failure insurance claim and, while the matter is being processed, a notice under the Act is served on the client; the subject matter of the notice might be linked to the claim, perhaps influencing its outcome; or

(c) The architect is acting for an owner who has been served a statutory notice and whose affected property contains occupiers; they, in accordance with the terms of their tenure require the protection of their landlord/owner; the architect has been asked to act as a party wall surveyor on the adjoining owner's behalf and also to act directly for those occupiers.

On the face of it, and in circumstances similar to those suggested above, the architect should carefully consider his position and, if at all possible, offer the appointment to a colleague who might be further distanced from the firm's client; if no such convenient compromise presents itself then to accept the appointment could present a conflict of interests and his impartiality may be open to question.

Irrespective of assurances of impartiality and blandishments that may be offered by the building owner's surveyor to his counterpart, it is obvious that for the surveyors to discharge their duties in an entirely unbiased way, in accordance with the requirements of the statute, the problems of agency and conflicts of interests must be dealt with at the outset.

Architects have traditionally had to deal with these problems with that degree of impartiality necessary to properly administer standard forms of building contract, and they are obliged to act in a neutral manner in the interests of both parties while still holding the balance between client and contractor in a fair and unbiased way.

Whether or not the architect's legal obligation to act impartially in his dealings with the parties to the contract can be considered analogous to that of the surveyor appointed under the provisions of the Party Wall etc. Act 1996 is debatable, but the notable difference is that an architect is employed by his client to administer a contract agreed between the client and the contractor while the party wall surveyor's appointment is one made under statute and is aimed to resolve a dispute between the parties.

Reality dictates that if architects acting as party wall surveyors do accept appointments in circumstances that might give rise to potential conflicts of interest then it is incumbent on them to maintain the unbiased manner normally required of an architect or of an agreed surveyor and to make every effort to be seen to be fair to all parties.

Architects and the Party Wall etc. Act 1996

13

It is therefore important that an architect should refuse an appointment to act as a party wall surveyor (and especially as an agreed surveyor) in situations where a conflict of interests might be generated.

Separate terms of engagement should be agreed between the architect and his client, the appointing owner, clearly citing the terms of his remit as a party wall surveyor and confirming his authority to act for the appointing owner in signing, issuing and receiving notices and making any necessary appointment on his behalf.

The Act requires all appointments and selections to be made and confirmed in writing, and as it is customary for each appointed surveyor to ask to see the other's letter of appointment to ensure that the appointments have been made in accordance with the terms of the Act. It is also prudent for the building owner's surveyor to have his fees agreed and confirmed in a separate letter.

Defining the party wall surveyor's role

It is important to understand and appreciate the scope of the remit of the appointed surveyor or surveyors, and defining its extent can give rise to differences of opinion. It has been suggested by a well-respected legal expert in the field that 'Firstly, the nature of the jurisdiction of party wall surveyors is that of experts. Their role is essentially technical, to design, approve and check the quality of the work with which they are concerned under Section 10. They are in no sense a tribunal. They are employed by the parties, or in the case of the third surveyor appointed by the party-appointed surveyors. It has never been considered that they are bound to act judicially or obliged to hold any sort of hearing before reaching a decision, or to give reasons. This view is reflected in the Chartered Society of Physiotherapy case. (*Party Walls – Law and Practice, 2nd Ed, 2004*, page 88.)

First, it should be noted that the third surveyor is not appointed but is selected, and the views expressed above are not shared by all, in that they are considered to be too broad as statements of the party wall surveyor's function to suggest that his role is that of a technical expert 'to design, approve and check the quality of the work with which they are concerned'.

The role of the surveyor under the Party Wall etc. Act 1996 must be construed in the light of Section 10; his role is to determine disputes and settle matters by the making of awards. It is of interest that a surveyor under the Act need have no formal qualifications at all and, reasonably, cannot be expected to be qualified in all possible disciplines such as architecture, structural engineering, quantity surveying, building surveying and project management, let alone, for example, in such technical specialisms as piling.

The surveyors' role is essentially quasi-arbitral and is concerned with the resolution of disputes between the parties. Disputes may turn upon a number of issues, and the surveyor's predominant role is to determine them and not to provide solutions to the disputed matters.

Thus the scope of Section 10(13) is sufficiently broad as to permit – as is not at all uncommon – awards to make appropriate provision for the costs of the various experts who may be consulted in the performance of the statutory function.

The party wall surveyors are not employed by the parties but, pursuant to statute, are appointed by them to perform a statutory function. That statutory function is not in the provision of expert opinion upon the subsidiary subject matter of disputes to which they are not parties but in the making of awards determining those disputes.

The suggestion that must be resisted is that party wall surveyors can in any controlling way be involved in designing, approving and checking the quality of the work with which they are 'concerned'.

The sense in which they are 'concerned' can only be with reference to the surveyor's role in considering and determining the nature of a building owner's proposal, its necessary compliance with the relevant sections of the statute, and whether or not the situation provides that a building owner may exercise his statutory rights; any other direct involvement by the surveyor in the design or formulation of the notifiable proposals would negate his neutral position and could be seen to be partisan.

As for 'approving and checking' the quality of the work, it must be understood that the party wall surveyor will make only those inspections necessary to ensure that the authorised work complies with the Act and the award. Should the building owner's work be found to be defective or unauthorised, it is for the building owner himself, usually through his consultants, to rectify the situation. The party wall surveyor has no remit to issue instructions and is not party to the dispute, although consequential disputed matters might be resolved by the making of an addendum award.

Sections 1–22
of the Party Wall Act,
discussed

Sections 1–22 of the Party Wall Act, discussed

Section 1 New building on line of junction

Section 1(1)(a), (b)

(1) This section shall have effect where lands of different owners adjoin and–

   (a) are not built on at the line of junction; or

   (b) are built on at the line of junction only to the extent of a boundary wall (not being a party fence wall or the external wall of a building),

   and either owner is about to build on any part of the line of junction.

Section 1, (1) to (8), concerns the proposal for new building on the line of junction of the lands of different owners where (1)(a) on that boundary line there is no existing structure, or where (1)(b) on the line of junction, the face of a boundary wall may denote the legal boundary when that wall is built entirely on the land of one of the owners and is in his sole ownership.

Section 1(2) and (3)(a), (b)

(2) If a building owner desires to build a party wall or party fence wall on the line of junction he shall, at least one month before he intends the building work to start, serve on any adjoining owner a notice which indicates his desire to build and describes the intended wall.

(3) If, having been served with notice described in subsection (2), an adjoining owner serves on the building owner a notice indicating his consent to the building of a party wall or party fence wall–

   (a) the wall shall be built half on the land of each of the two owners or in such other position as may be agreed between the two owners; and

   (b) the expense of building the wall shall be from time to time defrayed by the two owners in such proportion as has regard to the use made or to be made of the wall by each of them and to the cost of labour and materials prevailing at the time when that use is made by each owner respectively.

Before starting building operations, a building owner wishing to build a wall astride a boundary must serve notice on any adjoining owner, describing fully the work intended and the date it is to start on site. The notice must allow for at least one month to elapse from the date of service of the notice to the intended commencement date.

If the adjoining owner consents to the proposed work, he must give the building owner written confirmation to that effect within 14 days from the date of receipt of the notice.

Where a boundary wall exists on the line of junction, a new building may entail its demolition or incorporation into the new wall to be built partly on the adjoining owner's land. It is usual for the parties to agree to the new wall being built with half its width on the land of each owner. However, if site conditions make this impractical, the owners may agree to the wall being built eccentrically about the line of junction. When built astride the line of junction, the wall will be legally defined as a party wall or party fence wall.

The precise position of the centre line of a wall built on the line of junction will not be the determining factor in any apportionment of construction costs. Costs will be assessed on the value of the use made of the wall by each owner and the amount agreed by the parties.

At the time of its construction, the adjoining owner may have no use for the wall, in which case the building owner must construct it at his own expense. However, if at some later date the adjoining owner wishes to make use of the party wall, he must then reimburse the building owner a proportion of the expense of building the wall based on the cost of materials and the labour rates prevailing at the time that such use is made. The calculation is to be agreed between the parties, or if they cannot agree, by surveyors appointed under Section 10.

Before he makes any use of the party wall, the adjoining owner must once again serve a party structure notice on the building owner in accordance with the requirements of Section 2. In exercising his rights to use the wall the adjoining owner becomes the building owner for the purposes of the Act, and the recipient of the notice then becomes the adjoining owner. A notice is valid for 12 months from the day it was served, after which time it will expire. The right to carry out any work which is the subject of the notice will be void if it has not been started within the 12-month period.

On the expiry of that notice, any appointments of surveyors will lapse. If any new notice which generates a dispute is subsequently served, then surveyors will have to be appointed under Section 10.

Section 1(4)(a), (b)

(4) If, having been served with notice described in subsection (2), an adjoining owner does not consent under this subsection to the building of a party wall or party fence wall, the building owner may only build the wall–

(a) at his own expense; and

(b) as an external wall or a fence wall, as the case may be, placed wholly on his own land,

and consent under this subsection is consent by a notice served within the period of fourteen days beginning with the day on which the notice described in subsection (2) is served.

If within 14 days of serving notice on the adjoining owner, the building owner does not receive written consent to his proposal to build a party wall on the line of junction, he may, entirely at his own expense and on his own land, build an external wall to his proposed building or a fence wall.

Section 1(5), (6)

(5) If the building owner desires to build on the line of junction a wall placed wholly on his own land he shall, at least one month before he intends the building work to start, serve on any adjoining owner a notice which indicates his desire to build and describes the intended wall.

(6) Where the building owner builds a wall wholly on his own land in accordance with subsection (4) or (5) he shall have the right, at any time in the period which–

(a) begins one month after the day on which the notice mentioned in the subsection concerned was served, and

(b) ends twelve months after that day,

to place below the level of the land of the adjoining owner such projecting footings and foundations as are necessary for the construction of the wall.

If a building owner proposes to build, on the line of junction, a wall wholly on his land, he must, at least one month before he intends to start work on site, serve notice on any adjoining owner stating his intentions and describing the work that he intends to carry out. Above ground level, the wall has to be built entirely on his own land, but any necessary footings or simple concrete foundations below ground may project into the adjoining owner's land. The building owner can place such foundations any time within the 12-month period, beginning one month after the day that the notice was served.

The adjoining owner has no right to refuse to allow the building owner to project simple foundations over the boundary, but reinforced or 'special foundations' may not be placed on the adjoining owner's land without his written consent.

The description 'special foundations' is defined in Section 20, and the reference to 'an assemblage of beams or rods' employed to carry or distribute loads is significant. If the normal practice of using a lightweight steel mesh in the concrete foundation cannot be considered to be enhancement of its load-bearing characteristics or essential for its function, then the foundation will not be a 'special foundation'.

Section 1(7)

(7) Where the building owner builds a wall wholly on his own land in accordance with subsection (4) or (5) he shall do so at his own expense and shall compensate any adjoining owner and any adjoining occupier for any damage to his property occasioned by–

(a) the building of the wall;

(b) the placing of any footings or foundations placed in accordance with subsection (6).

When on the line of junction a building owner builds a wall wholly on his own land, and at his own expense, he is required to compensate the adjoining owner or occupier for any damage that occurs as a result. If foundations are placed over the boundary, it is very likely that the adjoining owner's land will be disturbed by excavations, and there could be interference with planting, paving or underground services and drains.

Section 1(8)

(8) Where any dispute arises under this section between the building owner and any adjoining owner or occupier it is to be determined in accordance with section 10.

Where disagreements arise between the owners they must be resolved in accordance with Section 10. The appointed surveyors will settle by award matters of compensation for disturbance, or the extent to which necessary foundations may be placed on the adjoining owner's land.

Reference is made to the line of junction or boundary line between adjoining lands, and it should be noted that the Act does not empower appointed surveyors to decide the position of the boundary. A boundary is a matter of legal title, and if its position is not obvious, or could be the subject of differing opinions, it may only be decided by agreement between the owners themselves. This might require the examination of title deeds, land registry documents and drawings, and even then the matter may not be resolved without recourse to the courts. It is essential that the position of the boundary is agreed before notices are served or building works are started.

Section 2 Repair etc. of party wall: rights of owner

Section 2(1), (2)(a)

(1) This section applies where lands of different owners adjoin and at the line of junction the said lands are built on or a boundary wall, being a party fence wall or the external wall of a building, has been erected.

(2) A building owner shall have the following rights–

    (a) to underpin, thicken or raise a party structure, a party fence wall, or an external wall which belongs to the building owner and is built against a party structure or party fence wall;

Regardless of the rights given to them in this Section, owners should be aware of the need to comply with other statutory legislation which could have a serious bearing on their proposals and might adversely influence, modify or prohibit work to or against a party wall or party structure.

For example, before starting work, an owner might need to obtain consents and permissions under planning law or building regulations or dispensation from landlords, head lessees or leaseholders. An application for planning permission might have its prospects of success diminished by the effect of an Article 4 Direction regulating proposals otherwise dealt with as permitted development, or by intended alterations to a listed building being a controversial issue in the proposals. There could be easements registered as charges on land registries or restrictive covenants which, if not lifted by agreement or by application to the Lands Tribunal, would be obstacles difficult or impractical to overcome. The amount of time spent trying to resolve these matters could seriously prejudice the commencement of work on site.

Ownership of the party wall or structure is not relevant to the rights of owners under Section 2. A party wall or party structure may be in the sole ownership of one owner, yet the other owner may use it as though it were his own.

Section 2(2)(e) allows the building owner to demolish a party structure which is not strong enough or high enough for his purposes and rebuild it to a greater or lesser height or thickness.

The building owner can exercise these rights provided he complies with the statutory requirements under Section 2(3) and (4), that he must make good any damage caused to the adjoining owner's property and, if required by the adjoining owner, build up any relevant flues and chimney stacks to such heights and in such materials as the owners agree. If they cannot agree, the matter must be resolved by surveyors appointed under Section 10. It often happens that chimney stacks and flues become redundant, so that, by agreement (and provided this complies with relevant planning restrictions or building regulations concerned with ventilation) they may be capped off or removed.

Section 2(2)(b)

> (b) to make good, repair, or demolish and rebuild, a party structure or party fence wall in a case where such work is necessary on account of defect or want of repair of the structure or wall;

The rights which the building owner has under this subsection in carrying out work necessary because of defects in a party wall or structure, and also when he has instituted work for his own purposes, are subject to the conditions in Section 2(3) and 2(4).

Here the building owner could expect from the adjoining owner a contribution to the cost of repairing the defective wall, the amount depending on the use that the adjoining owner makes of the wall.

Under these subsections, the building owner must bear the cost of any work carried out when exercising the right given to him in Section 2(2)(e), provided the work is not necessary as a result of defects (Section 2(2)(b)).

Section 2(2)(c)–(e)

> (c) to demolish a partition which separates buildings belonging to different owners but does not confirm with statutory requirements and to build instead a party wall which does so conform;
>
> (d) in the case of buildings connected by arches or structures over public ways or over passages belonging to other persons, to demolish the whole or part of such buildings, arches or structures which do not conform with statutory requirements and to rebuild them so that they do so conform:
>
> (e) to demolish a party structure which is of insufficient strength or height for the purposes of any intended building of the building owner and to rebuild it of sufficient strength or height for the said purposes (including rebuilding to a lesser height or thickness where the rebuilt structure is of sufficient strength and height for the purposes of any adjoining owner);

Many existing buildings do not comply, in whole or in part, with current legislation. These paragraphs allow:

(c) the demolition of a non-conforming partition that separates buildings in separate ownerships, and its reinstatement with a party wall that does comply;

(d) the demolition of all or parts of non-conforming buildings connected by arches or other structures over public ways or passages not in the ownership of either owner, and their rebuilding so that they do conform;

(e) the demolition and rebuilding of a party structure as required by the building owner in accordance with the provisions of Section 2(2)(m) and Section 11(7).

Section 2(8) states that a building or structure which, prior to this Act being passed, conformed to relevant statutes at the time it was erected is deemed to conform to current legislation. While there is no statutory requirement to rebuild a non-conforming building, a building owner wishing to carry out material alterations to part of a non-conforming structure may be required to bring the whole of the building or buildings into compliance with current building regulations. An example would be where the integrity of structural compartmentation or means of escape was prejudiced by the building owner's works. Any work carried out in these circumstances would be the responsibility of the building owner at his own cost.

It should be noted from Section 2(2)(e) that while a building owner may reduce the height and thickness of a party structure, any rebuilding will have to ensure that it is of sufficient strength and height for the purposes of the adjoining owner. These may include his use of the wall as an enclosing wall to his building.

Section 2(2)(f)–(j)

(f) to cut into a party structure for any purpose (which may be or include the purpose of inserting a damp proof course);

(g) to cut away from a party wall, party fence wall, external wall or boundary wall any footing or any projecting chimney breast, jamb or flue, or other projection on or over the land of the building owner in order to erect, raise or underpin any such wall or for any other purpose;

(h) to cut away or demolish parts of any wall or building of an adjoining owner overhanging the land of the building owner or overhanging a party wall, to the extent that it is necessary to cut away or demolish the parts to enable a vertical wall to be erected or raised against the wall or building of the adjoining owner;

(j) to cut into the wall of an adjoining owner's building in order to insert a flashing or other weather-proofing of a wall erected against that wall;

A building owner has the right to cut into a party structure for any purpose, for example to provide padstones or seating for beams, or to carry out toothing or bonding of walls. He may drill or cut into a party structure to insert a damp-proof course which will remain in situ for the full thickness of the party structure and may straddle the line of junction.

Although openings may be made in a party structure – perhaps in the course of repair works requiring needling or propping – no permanent openings are permitted in an otherwise imperforate wall.

Chimney breasts, jambs, flues, footings and foundations or gutters projecting onto or over the building owner's land may be cut off, and he may raise, build or underpin a wall on a line of junction. He must not carry out work to the detriment of the adjoining owner and must make good any damage caused by his work – see Section 2(5). If required, he must provide an alternative but complete reinstatement of working flues, and where necessary provide continuity of the means of rainwater disposal or drainage from the adjoining owner's property.

It may happen that a building owner erects an independent building adjacent to an adjoining owner's wall or building and wishes to bridge and weatherproof the nominal space between the structures. Although both buildings could be situated on the line of junction they might be separate from each other. In Section 2(2)(j) the right is given to cut into a wall of an independent building to insert a flashing or weathering. However, without the express permission of the adjoining owner, cutting into his independent wall for other purposes (except to tie in a party wall as allowed for in Section 2(2)(k)) would constitute trespass.

Section 2(2)(k)

(k) to execute any other necessary works incidental to the connection of a party structure with the premises adjoining it;

Following the demolition of a building, the party wall might need stabilising by reinforcing or augmenting its ties with the adjoining owner's existing building or new construction. In that case, allowance should be made for the usual settlement of new work. The building owner is also entitled to tie a party wall or structure to an independent building adjacent to it.

Other necessary work to do with connecting the party wall with adjoining premises can include the provision of flashings and adequate temporary or permanent weatherings, and protection where a party wall formerly enclosed by an owner's building becomes an external wall enclosing an adjoining owner's building.

Section 2(2)(l)–(n)

(l) to raise a party fence wall, or to raise such a wall for use as a party wall, and to demolish a party fence wall and rebuild it as a party fence wall or as a party wall;

(m) subject to the provisions of section 11(7), to reduce, or to demolish and rebuild, a party wall or party fence wall to–

(i) a height of not less than two metres where the wall is not used by an adjoining owner to any greater extent than a boundary wall; or

(ii) a height currently enclosed upon by the building of an adjoining owner;

(n) to expose a party wall or party structure hitherto enclosed subject to providing adequate weathering.

Here the right is given to demolish and rebuild a party fence wall and rebuild it as a party wall, or demolish and rebuild a party wall as a party fence wall. The new wall will be astride the boundary in a position agreed by the owners, and may be used as an enclosing wall to the building owner's new structure.

Section 2(3), (4)

(3) Where work mentioned in paragraph (a) of subsection (2) is not necessary on account of defect or want of repair of the structure or wall concerned, the right falling within that paragraph is exercisable–

    (a) subject to making good all damage occasioned by the work to the adjoining premises or to their internal furnishings and decorations; and

    (b) where the work is to a party structure or external wall, subject to carrying any relevant flues and chimney stacks up to such a height and in such materials as may be agreed between the building owner and the adjoining owner concerned or, in the event of dispute, determined in accordance with section 10;

    and relevant flues and chimney stacks are those which belong to an adjoining owner and either form part of or rest on or against the party structure or external wall.

(4) The right falling within subsection (2)(e) is exercisable subject to–

    (a) making good all damage occasioned by the work to the adjoining premises or to their internal furnishings and decorations; and

    (b) carrying any relevant flues and chimney stacks up to such a height and in such materials as may be agreed between the building owner and the adjoining owner concerned or, in the event of dispute, determined in accordance with section 10;

    and relevant flues and chimney stacks are those which belong to an adjoining owner and either form part of or rest on or against the party structure.

Unless work carried out under paragraphs (a) or (e) of Subsection 2(2) is necessitated to remedy a defect in the party wall or structure concerned, the building owner will be responsible for any repairs or making good to the party structure and adjacent areas, both externally and internally where damage has been occasioned by his work.

There might be chimney stacks and flues in a party structure, demolished together with the party structure itself when the requirement is that it be demolished and rebuilt; those flues belonging to the adjoining owner must be reinstated to a working condition if the adjoining owner so requires.

Should a dispute arise as to the construction, the materials to be used or perhaps the heights of the proposed reinstatement of the flues, the matters must be referred to the appointed surveyors to be determined in accordance with the provisions of Section 10.

Where the work to the party structure is necessitated by wants of repair or the remedy of defects, the applicable costs are to be apportioned between the owners in accordance with the provisions of Section 11(4).

Apart from traditional brick or masonry flues built into a party structure, there could be proprietary flues serving the adjoining owner's hot water and central heating boilers with flues traversing the full thickness of the party structure, emerging with terminals fixed on the building owner's side of the party structure and often expelling gases into the building owner's airspace.

While it is incumbent on the building owner to make good damage caused by his notifiable work, it is important to establish that the adjoining owner is entitled to retain the flues and terminals serving his building and that their legitimacy has been confirmed by agreement or without such agreement and, as is often the case when the locations of the terminals originally may have constituted a trespass, by allowing the adjoining owner to retain the status quo when he can prove the benefit of adverse possession.

Obviously if the flues and terminals do trespass and the adjoining owner has no legal entitlement to retain them in their extant positions the building owner may cut them off without having any responsibility for their reinstatement.

Section 2(5)

(5) Any right falling within subsection (2)(f), (g) or (h) is exercisable subject to making good all damage occasioned by the work to the adjoining premises or to their internal furnishings and decorations.

However minor the work required to cut into a party structure or to cut off parts of the structure projecting over the building owner's land it nevertheless may cause damage both externally and internally to the adjoining owner's premises and the building owner is obliged to make good the damage caused by his work.

Section 2(6)

(6) The right falling within subsection (2)(j) is exercisable subject to making good all damage occasioned by the work to the wall of the adjoining owner's building.

Inserting a flashing into an adjoining owner's property generally necessitates the prior cutting of chases into its masonry. The work should be undertaken with due care and attention, and the building owner is liable for any damage to the adjoining owner's property caused by his work.

The Act, in this subsection, refers only to the wall of the adjoining property and not to any of its internal parts, but the constraints of Sections 7(1) and (2) will be sufficient to protect the adjoining owner and his property in the event that the building owner acts unreasonably or that he causes damage such that he is obliged to make compensation to adjoining owners or occupiers.

Section 2(7)(a), (b)

The right falling within subsection (2)(m) is exercisable subject to–

(a) reconstructing any parapet or replacing an existing parapet with another one; or

(b) constructing a parapet where one is needed but did not exist before.

Where a party wall or party fence wall is reduced in height, any parapet demolished in the process must be reinstated at a height required by the adjoining owner and often above the height of the wall enclosed by his premises.

In circumstances where previously an adjoining property had no parapet but, by virtue of the change of construction brought about by the reduction in height of the party wall or party fence wall one might be needed, then the building owner must provide it.

Section 2(8)

For the purposes of this section a building or structure which was erected before the day on which this Act was passed shall be deemed to conform with statutory requirements if it conforms with the statutes regulating buildings or structures on the date on which it was erected.

This subsection concerns work to existing structures which were built before the provisions of this Act came into force and provides that should those structures have complied with the relevant legislation on the day that they were built, their construction is deemed to comply with the current legislation regulating the building owner's proposed work.

It is evident that, should the building owner's proposals interfere or modify the structure to an extent that would compromise the constructional integrity of the adjoining owner's premises and its deemed conformity with past or current legislation, then he is obliged to remedy the situation and pay the costs of any work required to put the structure into a condition such that it will comply.

Section 3 Party structure notices

Section 3(1)(a)–(c)

(1) Before exercising any right conferred on him by section 2 a building owner shall serve on any adjoining owner a notice (in this Act referred to as "a party structure notice") stating–

    (a) the name and address of the building owner;

    (b) the nature and particulars of the proposed work including, in cases where the building owner proposes to construct special foundations, plans, sections and details of construction of the special foundations together with reasonable particulars of the loads to be carried thereby; and

    (c) the date on which the proposed work will begin.

Before a building owner can exercise any of those rights conferred on him by Section 2, allowing him to carry out any of the 13 permitted building operations specified in that section, he must serve a party structure notice on any adjoining owner who will be affected by the proposed work. Any unauthorised works started on site prior to the service of a party structure notice would be unlawful and could be the subject of an adjoining owner making application to the courts for an injunction to stop them.

In instances where unauthorised works are advanced or even completed, and while an injunction could be sought to demolish them, the consequent burden of ensuing costs and expenses will almost certainly be placed on the building owner unless, for example, the adjoining owner having been made aware that the works were being progressed had omitted to halt them and had therefore condoned them by his inaction.

The party structure notice must be served on the adjoining owner(s) whose name and address must be correctly entered in the documents; the nature and particulars of the proposed works must be clearly stated so that the adjoining owner has sufficient information to decide to consent or dissent to the notice or perhaps, being given the opportunity, he may wish to serve on the building owner a counter notice requiring the building owner to carry out additional works for the adjoining owner's benefit.

Inaccuracies in the information given in the notice may lead to it being challenged and perhaps voided and could delay matters. The consequences of serving an invalid notice give rise to the procedures having to be started afresh with the building owner being required to reissue and serve an appropriate notice in a properly corrected form.

If the building owner wishes to construct special foundations and proposes to place them on the adjoining owner's land, he must provide the adjoining owner with any necessary plans, sections and details of their construction together with those of the superstructure and the loads that will be placed on them. A building owner has no right to construct special foundations on an adjoining owner's land without first obtaining from him express consent in writing to the proposals; an adjoining owner's unwillingness or refusal to give consent for special foundations does not constitute a disagreement or dispute that can be resolved under any of the provisions of the Act and the building owner has no right to trespass.

The building owner should be prepared to pay the costs likely to be incurred when the adjoining owner needs to give proper consideration to the technical issues arising from the building owner's wish to construct special foundations or other temporary enabling works on the adjoining land. To enable him to respond and perhaps give his consent to the building owner it would be prudent for the adjoining owner to obtain independent structural engineering advice as to the consequences of allowing the proposed work to be executed.

The building owner is obliged to give notice of two calendar months before the intended works can start on site and the party structure notice should be dated accordingly; it should be noted that the period of two calendar months begins not necessarily on the date stated on the notice but on the date on which the notice is served on the adjoining owner.

The building owner is not entitled to start the authorised works before time has run but to facilitate the building owner's programme the adjoining owner can give his written agreement to a period of time less than the statutory two months prescribed in the Act so as to attain an earlier date. In the event of a dispute arising necessitating the appointment of surveyors under the provisions of Section 10 a period of less than two months may be insufficient for obtaining the information necessary to make an award.

Section 3(2)(a), (b)(i), (ii)

(2) A party structure notice shall–

    (d) be served at least two months before the date on which the proposed work will begin;

    (e) cease to have effect if the work to which it relates–

        (i) has not begun within the period of twelve months beginning with the day on which the notice is served; and

        (ii) is not prosecuted with due diligence.

A party structure notice must be served at least two calendar months before notifiable work may start on site. The building owner must begin the work and diligently proceed with it within 12 months from the date of the service of notice on the adjoining owner or, if the matter has given rise to a dispute, at a date agreed in an award.

Diligently proceeding with the work requires that it should be carried out with continuity and without unnecessarily long periods of inactivity.

Notice will have expired if the work has not been started within the prescribed 12 months, and so, if the building owner still intends to do the work, he must serve a new notice. This will apply irrespective of the adjoining owner having given written consent to the original notice although, if the work had been started and is subject to an award, then the provisions of the award may apply.

Section 3(3)(a), (b)

(3) Nothing in this section shall–

  (a) prevent a building owner from exercising with the consent in writing of the adjoining owners and of the adjoining occupiers any right conferred on him by section 2; or

  (b) require a building owner to serve any party structure notice before complying with any notice served under any statutory provisions relating to dangerous or neglected structures.

If a building owner serves a party structure notice on an adjoining owner and obtains the adjoining owner's and occupiers' written consent both to the work described in the notice and to the waiver of the two-month period before work is permitted to start on site then the building owner may start the work immediately. It is important to note that under the Act occupiers are not entitled to receive notice of the building owner's proposals but nevertheless their written consent is required and has to be obtained by the adjoining owner so as to permit the building owner to start work before the expiration of the statutory period of notice.

There is no requirement for a building owner to serve a party structure notice on any adjoining owner when immediate and necessary repair or preservation works are required to stabilise his building; also, having to comply with the terms of a dangerous structure notice will supersede the requirement to serve a party structure notice.

Without giving notice, a building owner may not proceed to carry out work to a neglected structure unless the work is necessitated as a consequence of neglect to maintain its fabric (other than for minor cosmetic refurbishment or redecoration), and this neglect has caused, or is causing, it to become dangerous.

Section 4 Counter notices

Section 4(1)(a), (b)(i), (ii)

(1) An adjoining owner may, having been served with a party structure notice serve on the building owner a notice (in this Act referred to as a "counter notice") setting out–

    (a) in respect of a party fence wall or party structure, a requirement that the building owner build in or on the wall or structure to which the notice relates such chimney copings, breasts, jambs or flues, or such piers or recesses or other like works, as may reasonably be required for the convenience of the adjoining owner;

    (b) in respect of special foundations to which the adjoining owner consents under section 7(4) below, a requirement that the special foundations–

        (i) be placed at a specified greater depth than that proposed by the building owner; or

        (ii) be constructed of sufficient strength to bear the load to be carried by columns of any intended building of the adjoining owner,

    or both.

An adjoining owner in receipt of a notice under Section 3 may serve on a building owner a counter notice when he might wish to profit from the opportunity provided by the building owner to carry out works on the adjoining owner's behalf. The adjoining owner may have intended to do work to his own property and perhaps had planned them to be carried out at some future date, not concurrently with those of the building owner. The requested works would be entirely to the adjoining owner's advantage and extra to the building owner's own works. These might involve amendments or additions to the building owner's proposals and could include new or extended chimneys, breasts, jambs and flues, copings, piers or recesses.

If the adjoining owner consents, or had consented, to special foundations being placed on his land but with the requirement that they be made sufficiently strong for his own intended works and perhaps incorporating stronger foundations placed at a greater depths than those intended by the building owner, the adjoining owner would be liable for the additional costs arising from the required changes to the building owner's original proposals.

A counter notice must be served on the building owner by the adjoining owner; if he has dissented from the building owner's original notice and has appointed a surveyor to act in the matter then the surveyor, if expressly authorised by his letter of appointment from the adjoining owner, may serve the notice on the adjoining owner's behalf.

Section 4(2)(a), (b)

(2) A counter notice shall–

    (a) specify the works required by the notice to be executed and shall be accompanied by plans, sections and particulars of such works; and

    (b) be served within the period of one month beginning with the day on which the party structure notice is served.

Section 4(3)(a)–(c)

(3) A building owner on whom a counter notice has been served shall comply with the requirements of the counter notice unless the execution of the works required by the counter notice would–

    (a) be injurious to him;

    (b) cause unnecessary inconvenience to him; or

    (c) cause unnecessary delay in the execution of the works pursuant to the party structure notice.

A counter notice must be served within one month following the adjoining owner's receipt of the building owner's original notice.

The counter notice must provide the building owner with comprehensive specifications and accurate detailed drawings of the adjoining owner's proposals in order that the building owner may be able to consider the consequences of complying with the adjoining owner's requirements.

For the adjoining owner's requested works to be accepted for incorporation into the building owner's programme they would have to be of a relatively simple nature and their implementation cannot be allowed to present the building owner with serious technical difficulties should he agree to carry them out. If a counter notice would unnecessarily inconvenience or injuriously affect the building owner or cause his works to be unnecessarily delayed he need not comply with the adjoining owner's request.

Section 5 Disputes arising under Sections 3 and 4

If an owner on whom a party structure notice or a counter notice has been served does not serve a notice indicating his consent to it within the period of fourteen days beginning with the day on which the party structure notice or counter notice was served, he shall be deemed to have dissented from the notice and a dispute shall be deemed to have arisen between the parties.

Within 14 days from the day that a building owner receives a counter notice from an adjoining owner he must serve on the adjoining owner written consent to the subject matter of the counter notice. Should the building owner wish to dissent from the notice or should he neglect to respond to it, a dispute is deemed to have arisen between the parties and the matter must be resolved by the appointment of surveyors under the provisions of Section 10.

Section 6 Adjacent excavation and construction

Section 6(1)(a), (b)

(1) This section applies where–

    (a) a building owner proposes to excavate, or excavate for and erect a building or structure, within a distance of three metres measured horizontally from any part of a building or structure of an adjoining owner; and

    (b) any part of the proposed excavation, building or structure will within those three metres extend to a lower level than the level of the bottom of the foundations of the building or structure of the adjoining owner.

A building owner intending to excavate, or excavate and build, within 3 m of the foundations of an adjoining owner's building must serve notice on the owner if any part of the intended excavations will extend below the bottom of the foundations of the adjoining owner's building. The wording of the section makes it clear that this applies to any excavation, regardless of whether or not it is a prelude to construction works.

For example, investigative trial holes might be needed to establish the nature and depths of adjacent foundations and may have to be dug deeper than the foundations. Soil test bores are also excavations, although they rarely have a material effect on adjacent structures. However, if there could be a potential for damage, it would be wise to serve notice.

Section 6(2)(a), (b)

(2) This section also applies where–

(a) a building owner proposes to excavate, or excavate for and erect a building or structure, within a distance of six metres measured horizontally from any part of a building or structure of an adjoining owner; and

(b) any part of the proposed excavation, building or structure will within those six metres meet a plane drawn downwards in the direction of the excavation, building or structure of the building owner at an angle of forty-five degrees to the horizontal from the line formed by the intersection of the plane of the level of the bottom of the foundations of the building or structure of the adjoining owner with the plane of the external face of the external wall of the building or structure of the adjoining owner.

There may be instances where more than one adjacent building could be affected. The building owner is required to give notice to any adjoining owner if he intends to excavate within 6 m of an adjacent building and where, within that horizontal distance, any part of his proposed excavations or building (piles) would cut a line drawn at 45° from the intersection of a downward projected line of the face of the adjacent building with the line of the bottom of its foundations.

The 6 m is measured from the nearest part of the adjacent building – usually its footings or foundations – to the nearest part of the building owner's excavation or building, foundation or piles.

Section 6(3), (4)

(3) The building owner may, and if required by the adjoining owner shall, at his own expense underpin or otherwise strengthen or safeguard the foundations of the building or structure of the adjoining owner so far as may be necessary.

(4) Where the buildings or structures of different owners are within the respective distances mentioned in subsections (1) and (2) the owners of those buildings or structures shall be deemed to be adjoining owners for the purposes of this section.

The proposed works might affect the foundations of the adjoining owner's building to the extent where these might need underpinning, strengthening or safeguarding. If the adjoining owner requires this, the building owner must carry out whatever work is agreed to be appropriate and necessary. If the need to carry out such precautionary work is disputed by either owner, matters must be resolved under Section 10, and any work to be carried out to the foundations of the adjoining owner's building, resulting from the excavations, will be at the building owner's sole expense.

In Section 6(4) the definition of 'adjoining owner' is not limited to an owner whose building or land immediately adjoins the building owner's land. An owner whose building is within the distances specified in Section 6(1) and 6(2) but does not immediately adjoin it, may be defined as an adjoining owner. This might be the case where, for example, there is an intervening property or a road belonging to a third party between the building owner's and the adjoining owner's properties. If there is a building or structure on the intervening land, the owner may also be an adjoining owner. In these circumstances each adjoining owner is entitled to be given notice of the proposals.

Section 6(5), (6)

(5) In any case where this section applies the building owner shall, at least one month before beginning to excavate, or excavate for and erect a building or structure, serve on the adjoining owner a notice indicating his proposals and stating whether he proposes to underpin or otherwise strengthen or safeguard the foundations of the building or structure of the adjoining owner.

(6) The notice referred to in subsection (5) shall be accompanied by plans and sections showing–

　(a) the site and depth of any excavation the building owner proposes to make;

　(b) if he proposes to erect a building or structure, its site.

In any of the situations provided for in Section 6(5), a building owner wishing to carry out excavation, or excavation and building works, is obliged to serve notice on any adjoining owner at least one month before he proposes to commence operations on site. The notice must provide full details of the proposals and be accompanied by plans and sections showing the siting and depth of the excavations and the siting of any proposed building or structure. It must state whether the building owner proposes to underpin or otherwise strengthen or safeguard the foundations of the adjoining owner's building in sufficient detail to enable the adjoining owner to decide whether underpinning will be needed. A notice is invalid if it does not give the precise information required by the Act.

Section 6(7)

(7) If an owner on whom a notice referred to in subsection (5) has been served does not serve a notice indicating his consent to it within the period of fourteen days beginning with the day on which the notice referred to in subsection (5) was served, he shall be deemed to have dissented from the notice and a dispute shall be deemed to have arisen between the parties.

Within 14 days of receiving notice, the adjoining owner must reply in writing saying that he agrees to the building owner's proposals. If he does not give written consent within 14 days, he is deemed to have dissented from the notice and the dispute must be resolved in accordance with Section 10.

If for some reason an adjoining owner fails to reply within the statutory period and is therefore deemed to have dissented by default, it is still possible to change that dissent to consent, provided that the adjoining owner agrees. This would void the appointment of any surveyors already appointed as a consequence of a deemed dissent.

Section 6(8)

(8) The notice referred to in subsection (5) shall cease to have effect if the work to which the notice relates–

    (a) has not begun within the period of twelve months beginning with the day on which the notice was served; and

    (b) is not prosecuted with due diligence.

As with party structure notices, a notice ceases to have effect if the work to which it relates has not been started within 12 months from the day it was served, or was not properly progressed within the 12-month period. Although the Act allows 12 months for the building owner to start on site and proceed diligently with his works, the owners may amend these dates and arrangements as they wish. However, even when notices are served and awards finalised in strict compliance with legislation, the start of building operations is often delayed for unforeseen reasons. In that event, to avoid having to serve new notices and appoint surveyors all over again, owners should try to agree revised dates and the adjoining owner be asked for written consent to waive notice.

Section 6(9)

(9) On completion of any work executed in pursuance of this section the building owner shall if so requested by the adjoining owner supply him with particulars including plans and sections of the work.

In most building contracts the completed works will contain minor variations from the details set out in the drawings and specifications both in the notices and in the award. Minor variations agreed by the owners, or by the appointed surveyors on their behalf, should be noted on 'as built' plans, sections and specifications and be supplied to the adjoining owner on request.

Figure 1 Application of 6 m and 3 m notices

Section 6 of the Act refers to the notices required in the event that the Building Owner proposes to carry out excavation or construction within a distance of 3 m or 6 m from an Adjoining Owner's building.

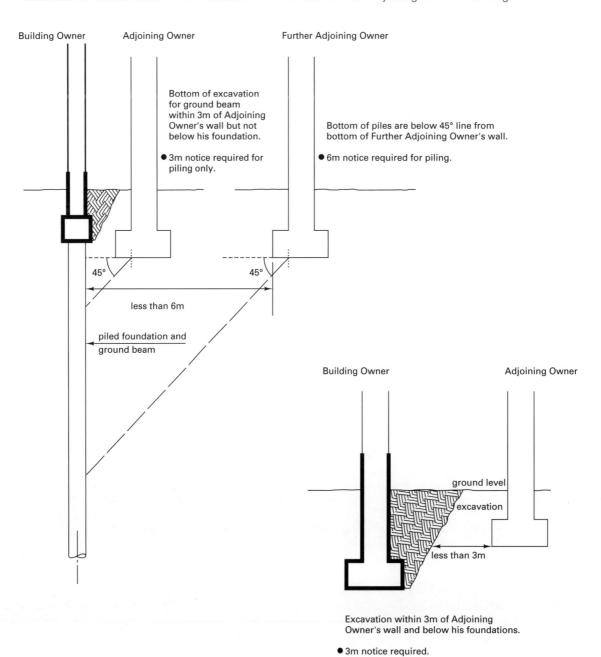

Building Owner   Adjoining Owner   Further Adjoining Owner

Bottom of excavation for ground beam within 3m of Adjoining Owner's wall but not below his foundation.

● 3m notice required for piling only.

Bottom of piles are below 45° line from bottom of Further Adjoining Owner's wall.

● 6m notice required for piling.

45°   45°

less than 6m

piled foundation and ground beam

Building Owner   Adjoining Owner

ground level

excavation

less than 3m

Excavation within 3m of Adjoining Owner's wall and below his foundations.

● 3m notice required.

Section 6(10)

(10) Nothing in this section shall relieve the building owner from any liability to which he would otherwise be subject for injury to any adjoining owner or any adjoining occupier by reason of work executed by him.

Whether or not an award has been settled, and in spite of the fact that the adjoining owner consented to the building owner's works, nothing relieves the building owner of his personal liability for injury sustained by an adjoining owner or occupier as a consequence of the execution of his works.

Section 6 of the Act refers to the notices required in the event that the building owner proposes to carry out excavation or construction within a distance of 3 m or 6 m from an adjoining owner's building.

Section 7 Rights etc.

Section 7(1)

(1) A building owner shall not exercise any right conferred on him by this Act in such a manner or at such time as to cause unnecessary inconvenience to any adjoining owner or to any adjoining occupier.

It is to be expected that building works to a party wall, or excavation works being carried out, near or close to an adjoining or adjacent property and within the horizontal distances defined in Section 6 of the Act will usually affect adjoining owners and occupiers and cause them some inconvenience and disruption. This section provides for the protection of adjoining owners and occupiers in those circumstances but also imposes a duty on the building owner to observe the provisions and constraints of other relevant legislation concerned with environmental health and noise pollution. Equally he must refrain from causing unnecessary inconvenience although in exercising his conferred rights such inconvenience caused by the works is, by the physical nature of the works themselves, often necessary and unavoidable.

What establishes 'necessary' inconvenience is to be decided on the facts of the matter which may, if not agreed by the owners, give rise to a deemed or an actual dispute necessitating determination and award by the appointed surveyors.

In the circumstances of the adjoining owner having consented to the building owner's proposals but not having agreed to the manner in which the building owner intends to carry them out a dispute arises, and it is required that the matter be resolved by surveyors acting under the provisions of Section 10. The building owner wishing to proceed in a way to which the adjoining owner cannot agree may consider that the inconvenience he causes is justified but he has to be reasonable and not be in breach of the provisions of Subsection (1) of this section. In resolving the dispute the surveyors may agree to award that an alternative way of working might obviate, as far as is practical, any unnecessary inconvenience but allow for a measure of unavoidable inconvenience so as to permit the building owner to proceed with the works while still giving due consideration to the wellbeing of adjoining owners and occupiers.

Section 7(2)

(2) The building owner shall compensate any adjoining owner and any adjoining occupier for any loss or damage which may result to any of them by reason of any work executed in pursuance of this Act.

The Act does not confer any right to cause unnecessary inconvenience to an adjoining owner, tenant or occupier in return for compensation.

Inconvenience caused by noise, vibration, dust etc. may all be generally associated with building works, but an example of unnecessary inconvenience might be the building owner's contractors unreasonably delaying the progress of the works – and it would be no defence for the building owner to claim that the delay was not of his making but was the fault of his contractors and that they were liable for the breach of the duty imposed on him by the provisions of Section 7. A serious breach of the building owner's duty would give grounds for a claim for damages being brought against him.

The Act does not provide for the appointed surveyors themselves to determine, by award, an adjoining owner's claim either for breach of statutory duty or for 'damage for nuisance', because the resolution of such claims falls outside their remit; they have no power to resolve matters that are properly dealt with by the courts. There is no provision in the Act for the appointed surveyors to award damages by way of compensation but they are, as an example, able to award compensation by way of payment 'assessed as a fair allowance' Section 11(6) for any inconvenience, necessary or otherwise, caused by the building owner exercising his rights under the provisions of Section 2(2)(e).

Compensation is payable to an adjoining owner for any loss or damage that he has suffered as a consequence of the building owner's authorised works. Initially it is for the owners to agree the particulars of any due compensation, and this is to be assessed on the extent of loss or damage caused and the cost of its rectifications or, alternatively, the adjoining owner can opt for a financial settlement in lieu of the building owner carrying out repairs. If the owners cannot agree, it is for the appointed surveyors to determine and award accordingly.

Directly resulting from works executed in pursuance of the Act and in addition to those specifically relating to loss or damage 'to property' (Section 1(7)), any form of loss suffered by the adjoining owner or occupier can be the subject of compensation and could include for loss of trade or interference with business on the adjoining owner's land, or it could be concerned with the difference in the market value of his property as calculated before and after the execution of the authorised works.

Section 7(3)

> (3) Where a building owner in exercising any right conferred on him by this Act lays open any part of the adjoining land or building he shall at his own expense make and maintain so long as may be necessary a proper hoarding, shoring or fans or temporary construction for the protection of the adjoining land or building and the security of any adjoining occupier.

Where a building owner wishes to exercise his right, for example, to demolish and rebuild a party fence wall or party wall, Section 2(2)(b)–(e), the physical act of opening up of parts of the adjoining owner's land or structure is referred to as 'laying open' and he will be required to provide, for as long as is necessary, temporary screens, hoardings, shoring, temporary constructions and fans in order to safeguard the adjoining owner's land and buildings and to protect any adjoining occupiers from hazard.

The potentially damaging effects of laying open an adjoining property become even more problematical if the property is occupied. The cost of carrying out the authorised works will generally be substantial and will most certainly be increased when added to the costs generated from any necessary negotiations concerning access required for the execution of the work, methods of protection for the adjoining property or the settlement of compensation claims made by interested and affected adjoining owners or occupiers.

The necessity can arise for the destruction of specific shared parts of a structure and often can be related to the maintenance of listed buildings where, to avoid its demolition and reinstatement, every viable alternative should be examined before the adjoining building is laid open. Nevertheless repair or reconstruction works may be unavoidable and sometimes arrive as a consequence of a building owner having been served a dangerous structure notice or other statutory notice requiring urgent remedial action to be taken to limit the possibility of damage occurring or even, in extreme cases, structural collapse.

Where the demolition of a semi-detached property is to be carried out to allow for redevelopment, it is usual to design a proposed new building so that its layout does not require the laying open of the adjoining structure. To maximise the site coverage of the new building by fully occupying the available land to the centre line of the party wall would necessitate laying open, but the preferred option is to leave the extant party wall in situ where it will abut the new development, and any fixings of the new works to the party wall are to be in accordance with the provisions of Section 2(2)(f), (g) and (k).

Underpinning of the foundations of an old party wall will usually be required when a new building is positioned against it; it should be noted that party walls in old buildings are rarely found to be plumb, and due allowance should be made for this when setting out the proposed adjacent building.

Section 7(4)

(4) Nothing in this Act shall authorise the building owner to place special foundations on land of an adjoining owner without his previous consent in writing.

Special foundations are defined in Section 20 as 'foundations in which an assemblage of beams or rods is employed for the purpose of distributing any load'. This description includes foundations comprised of grillages of steel beams encased in concrete or, more usually, reinforced concrete.

A building owner wishing to place special foundations on adjoining land must first obtain the adjoining owner's written consent to the proposal because without this his only option would be to construct the foundations entirely on his own land. Placing special foundations on adjoining land could have considerable monetary implications for a building owner and possibly his successors in title should the adjoining owner's land be developed at some future date and long after the special foundations had been placed – see Section 11(10).

Section 7(5)(a), (b)

(5) Any works executed in pursuance of this Act shall–

(a) comply with the provisions of statutory requirements; and

(b) be executed in accordance with such plans, sections and particulars as may be agreed between the owners or in the event of dispute determined in accordance with section 10;

and no deviation shall be made from those plans, sections and particulars except such as may be agreed between the owners (or surveyors acting on their behalf) or in the event of dispute determined in accordance with section 10.

It is unlawful for a building owner to carry out works subject to notice before obtaining the adjoining owner's written consent to the proposals. The intended works must comply with all relevant statutory requirements and must be carried out in strict accordance with plans, sections and other necessary particulars to be agreed between the parties. In default of such agreement, work is not to be executed without the authority of an award that states the required terms and conditions to be observed in accordance with the provisions of Section 10.

Following a change of plan or perhaps due to changes in site conditions it might become necessary for the owners, or the surveyors acting on their behalf, to agree variations or amendments on the subject detail of the original agreement.

If the parties are unable to agree the variations, the disputed matters must again be determined under the provisions of Section 10.

It is important to note that other than for agreement to variations of a minor nature, neither the owners nor the appointed surveyors have authority to agree any material variation that could affect or alter the details of works given in the building owner's original notice and that would necessitate, in regard to any changed nature of the proposed works, the service of a new notice.

Section 8 Rights of entry

Section 8(1)

> (1) A building owner, his servants, agents and workmen may during usual working hours enter and remain on any land or premises for the purpose of executing any work in pursuance of this Act and may remove any furniture or fittings or take any other action necessary for that purpose.

This important subsection confers on the building owner the right to enter an adjoining owner's land during normal working hours for the specific purpose of carrying out work which is the subject of notice under Sections 1, 2 or 6; his servants and employees, his appointed surveyor, his agents and workmen may also, together with their tools and equipment, enter and remain on the adjoining property for as long as necessary to complete the work.

Fitted furniture and fixtures such as cupboards and other similar units located in the area of the proposed work may cause obstruction but only if it is entirely necessary may they be removed from the adjoining owner's premises to enable free access for the building owner's works.

Scaffolding, once erected, may be allowed to remain on adjoining land for all of the time necessary to carry out the authorised work, and during this period it may be modified and adjusted as required.

Normal working hours are usually from 08:30 to 18:00 on weekdays and 08:30 to 13:00 on Saturdays, and it is generally accepted that no work is permitted on Sundays and public holidays; working hours are regulated also by the local authority.

The proposed work must be held to be in pursuance of the Act, and will usually be defined in an award – see Subsections 7(5)(a), (b). The building owner is not entitled to claim the right of entry to carry out any unrelated or ancillary work without the express consent of the adjoining owner, and occupation of adjoining land for the purpose of carrying out unauthorised work without such consent will constitute trespass.

Other than for the execution of work in pursuance of the Act there is no right given or implied in Section 8 to permit, for example, entry onto adjoining land for the purpose of excavating trial holes to ascertain the depths of the foundations of adjoining buildings. A building owner wishing to know if he is required to serve notice of his proposals under the provisions of Section 6 needs specific information concerning the nature and depths of the foundations of the adjoining owner's property and, should access to the adjoining premises be denied, is very much disadvantaged if the requirement cannot be established.

A building owner intending to proceed with his work without the benefit of having full knowledge of the foundation depths of the adjoining property may nevertheless consider it expedient to serve a notice under the provisions of Section 6. The consequences of serving a notice which may later be found to have been unnecessary will be costly, but it would be prudent to ensure that the notice allows for the possibility of the adjoining building having a basement or foundations within the prescribed horizontal distances from the building owner's proposed work and at a higher level than its proposed foundations.

Section 8(2)

(2) If the premises are closed, the building owner, his agents and workmen may, if accompanied by a constable or other police officer, break open any fences or doors in order to enter the premises.

In the circumstances of adjoining premises being closed, i.e. locked or otherwise secured, and after all normal lawful attempts to gain entry have been unsuccessful, a building owner, his agents and workmen may, accompanied by a police officer, break down doors or destroy locks, barriers or fences in order to gain entry.

It is rare that a building owner needs to involve the police in these matters, but urgent necessity or an emergency could require him to take such extreme action. The building owner will be initially responsible for any damage caused in the attempts to gain entry, and the event should be carefully recorded; issues arising from it would normally be resolved by surveyors appointed under the provisions of Section 10.

Section 8(3)(a), (b)

(3) No land or premises may be entered by any person under subsection (1) unless the building owner serves on the owner and the occupier of the land or premises–

(a) in case of emergency, such notice of the intention to enter as may be reasonably practicable;

(b) in any other case, such notice of the intention to enter as complies with subsection (4).

Due written notice of the intention to enter adjoining premises must be given to adjoining owners and occupiers. Even though an emergency may not allow time for a building owner to serve the required minimum notice of at least 14 days, he must nevertheless give a detailed description of the nature of the work to be urgently undertaken and give as much notice as is possible and practicable in the circumstances prevailing.

Section 8(4)

Notice complies with this subsection if it is served in a period of not less than fourteen days ending with the day of the proposed entry.

Further to the service of written notice on any adjoining owner or occupier a period of not less than 14 days, to include the day of the proposed entry, must elapse before entry onto adjoining premises can be lawfully effected.

Section 8(5)

(5) A surveyor appointed or selected under section 10 may during usual working hours enter and remain on any land or premises for the purpose of carrying out the object for which he is appointed or selected.

It should be noted that this subsection refers to a surveyor being appointed or selected under Section 10, and provides that the appointed surveyors, as well as the selected third surveyor, may enter and remain on any relevant land or premises if that is what is considered necessary for them to carry out the object for which they are appointed or selected. The object for which the surveyors are appointed or selected is the determination of issues arising when work executed in pursuance of the Act is subject to dispute between the owners. A practical example of the consequences of an adjoining owner's refusal to allow access, perhaps for taking a necessary schedule of condition, might be when the surveyors make an award to extend their right of entry solely for that specific purpose.

Section 8(6)(a), (b)

(6) No land or premises may be entered by a surveyor under subsection (5) unless the building owner who is a party to the dispute concerned serves on the owner and the occupier of the land or premises–

(a) in case of emergency, such notice of the intention to enter as may be reasonably practicable;

(b) in any other case, such notice of the intention to enter as complies with subsection (4).

Before surveyors can enter on any land or premises belonging to either of the parties in dispute it is mandatory to serve notice of proposed entry on both owners and occupiers. The 'building owner' in the context of this subsection remains the owner who has served the notice (as in Section 10) that gives rise to the dispute, although it might be construed that the 'building owner' is the owner requiring right of entry for the surveyor he has appointed. Subsection 8(6) refers to the 'building owner who is a party to the dispute concerned' and, although both owners are party to the dispute, it is only the building owner who has given notice under Section 10.

A surveyor appointed under the provisions of Section 10 cannot, by either party to the dispute, be denied access to any relevant land and premises for the purpose of carrying out the object for which he is appointed, irrespective of which of the parties has appointed him – see Section 8(5). In the event that the building owner's surveyor is refused access to the adjoining owner's premises, the building owner can invoke the provisions of Section 8(6) by complying with the requirements of Section 8(4) and serving a notice of proposed entry.

Notice of proposed entry may only be served by the building owner (as in Section 10) who is a party to the dispute; a similar right is not conferred on the adjoining owner. If appointed surveyors are refused entry onto the building owner's premises, they may determine by award that the obstruction by the building owner is unlawful, that access must be provided and, in default, rely on the criminal sanctions set out in Section 16.

Section 9 Easements

Nothing in this Act shall–

  (a) authorise any interference with an easement of light or other easements in or relating to a party wall; or

  (b) prejudicially affect any right of any person to preserve or restore any right or other thing in or connected with a party wall in case of the party wall being pulled down or rebuilt.

The building owner's proposed works may affect established easements concerned with rights of light relating to a party wall or some other parts of an adjoining owner's premises and this is sometimes unavoidable.

Necessary and required work to a party wall will sometimes involve the exercising of rights conferred by Section 2(2)(a), (c) and (l) of the Act, and by others that give a building owner the right to demolish a party wall or party fence wall and rebuild it. Executing these works can interfere with the adjoining premises to an extent that could be prejudicial to its right to light. The right to rebuild a party wall, not necessarily to the original height prior to demolition but to a greater height required for the building owner's purposes cannot be exercised if it would physically extinguish a right to light or would result in the material diminution of light to adjoining premises.

In this context, therefore, any necessary interference with an adjoining owner's rights is not permitted to be other than of a temporary nature and is only allowed for that reasonable period of time to enable a building owner, without hindrance, to carry out authorised work. The right to an easement that has not ended by abandonment but perhaps has been overridden during the progress of the building operations must be reinstated immediately following the completion of the work.

A building may acquire an easement either by grant or prescription.

Subsection (a) is predominately concerned with the protection of easements of light, but other easements could include easements of support or easements of access and rights of way.

It can be difficult to obtain historical evidence sufficient to establish that an easement, if acquired, was either by grant or by prescription. It would be reasonable to allow for the investigation of deeds and the examination of written agreements made between the parties or previous holders of title, or from information gained from searching archives of the Land Registry or the local authority.

Subsection (b) provides that if an easement, perhaps a right to light, existed in a party wall that is later demolished and rebuilt, the reinstatement of the easement is allowed so far as it does not conflict with other relevant legislation governing permitted openings in new party wall construction.

Easements giving rights of support can be acquired by grant or gained by a building enjoying support from an adjoining building for an unbroken period of at least 20 years.

Continuing support may be adversely affected by demolition work lawfully carried out in pursuance of the Act but which may involve removal of adjoining buildings and exposure of party walls to the elements, and may cause the drying out of adjacent uncovered soil and subject shallow foundations to potential subsidence.

The necessity for the continuation of the right of support must be maintained and although reasonable interference with this right is permitted during the execution of authorised work, a building owner is liable to make good any damage it causes, in accordance with the provisions of Section 2(3)(a), (4)(a), (5), (6) and 7(2).

In dealing with the potential effects that easements could have on the implementation of authorised work, difficult problems might arise which require a specialised knowledge of the legalities concerned in disputed matters. While the remit of appointed surveyors does extend to allowing them to determine the issues in this specialist area and to award as necessary, it is accepted that they might need to seek professional advice and assistance from the appropriate legal authorities.

Section 10 Resolution of disputes

Section 10(1)(a), (b)

(1) Where a dispute arises or is deemed to have arisen between a building owner and an adjoining owner in respect of any matter connected with any work to which this Act relates either–

    (a) both parties shall concur in the appointment of one surveyor (in this section referred to as an "agreed surveyor"); or

    (b) each party shall appoint a surveyor and the two surveyors so appointed shall forthwith select a third surveyor (all of whom are in this section referred to as "the three surveyors").

Where a dispute arises, or is deemed to have arisen, surveyors must be appointed to resolve matters. The Act does not provide that owners may act for themselves in resolving the dispute (see definition of 'surveyor' in Section 20), and they must either concur in the appointment of a single surveyor, the 'agreed surveyor', or must each separately appoint a surveyor.

It is generally the case that where proposed notifiable work is relatively straightforward and uncomplicated, it would be the preferred option to choose the appointment of the 'agreed surveyor' as very often he would be better able to progress matters without having the delays in communication that occur between surveyors or the owners' consultants and, of course, incidental costs can be reduced considerably.

In the event that the owners each appoint a surveyor, it is for the two surveyors to immediately select a third surveyor, someone who can be called on to decide issues on which the appointed surveyors may disagree. The third surveyor does not need to know of his selection until such time as contention or a disagreement arises to make it necessary for the appointed surveyors, or either of the parties to the dispute, to request his intervention.

After being appointed by an adjoining owner a surveyor should immediately notify the building owner of this appointment so as to avoid the possibility of the building owner, not otherwise knowing of the appointment, serving notice on the adjoining owner under the provisions of Section 10(4) which would result in the building owner himself making the appointment of the adjoining owner's surveyor.

It is important to note that there is no requirement to appoint surveyors if an adjoining owner gives consent to the served notice; giving his consent does not deprive him of any entitlement to future protection of the Act, and disputed claims for compensation or for repairing damage occasioned by the building owner's work will themselves necessitate the appointment of surveyors.

Section 10(2)

> (2) All appointments and selections made under this section shall be in writing and shall not be rescinded by either party.

As for notices, all appointments must be made in writing.

The appointment of a surveyor is made under statute, is personal to the named surveyor and cannot be made of a company with which he might be associated or of a practice that employs him; his appointment can only be altered subject to the provisions of Section 10(3), (5) and (9).

Section 10(3)(a)–(d)

> (3) If an agreed surveyor–
>
> (a) refuses to act;
>
> (b) neglects to act for a period of ten days beginning with the day on which either party serves a request on him;
>
> (c) dies before the dispute is settled; or
>
> (d) becomes or deems himself incapable of acting, the proceedings for settling such dispute shall begin *de novo*.

An agreed surveyor is bound to carry out his duties in accordance with the terms of his appointment made under the provisions of this section of the Act but should he:

(a) refuse to act when action is necessary and required; or

(b) neglect to act for a period of ten days from the day he was served with a request to act; or

(c) die before the matter in dispute is resolved; or

(d) become incapable of acting due to matters beyond his control – for example those concerning illness or disability – or he might deem himself incapable of acting when the circumstances that prevailed when he accepted his appointment materially alter so as to make the continuation of the appointment in some aspect contrary to the provisions of the Act, the procedures for the resolution of the dispute must be started anew.

Section 10(4)(a), (b)

(4) If either party to the dispute–

    (a) refuses to appoint a surveyor under subsection (1)(b), or

    (b) neglects to appoint a surveyor under subsection (1)(b) for a period of ten days beginning with the day on which the other party serves a request on him,

the other party may make the appointment on his behalf.

The parties to the dispute are obliged to appoint surveyors immediately the dispute arises, but should either of the parties:

(a) refuse to appoint a surveyor as provided for in Subsection 10(1)(b); or

(b) not appoint a surveyor under Subsection 10(1)(b) and neglects so to do for a period of ten days from the day on which he was served with a request by the other party to make such appointment, the other party may make the appointment on his behalf.

It is necessary to adhere to the time constraints and procedures governing the appointment of surveyors so as to ensure compliance with provisions of the Act. Ignorance of the procedures or an unwillingness to follow them by either of the parties to the dispute must not be allowed to impede the progress of its resolution.

A party to the dispute may appoint a surveyor to act on behalf of the other party if, for any reason, a formal request to the other party has not achieved the obligatory statutory appointment.

On a construction site, there might be several adjoining owners and perhaps one who might default by not appointing a surveyor. When it becomes necessary that the building owner makes the appointment, the preferred choice would be of a surveyor who perhaps is familiar with the continuing project and has already been appointed by another adjoining owner. It is advisable that in these circumstances the building owner's choice of surveyor should be seen to clearly demonstrate the surveyor's independence in dealing with the matters for which he is appointed and that he has equal concern for the welfare of all parties to the dispute.

Section 10(5)

(5) If, before the dispute is settled, a surveyor appointed under paragraph (b) of subsection (1) by a party to the dispute dies, or becomes or deems himself incapable of acting, the party who appointed him may appoint another surveyor in his place with the same power and authority.

If, before a dispute is settled, a surveyor appointed under the provisions of Subsection 10(1)(b) dies or becomes incapable of acting, or deems himself incapable of acting, then it is important to note that only the party that appointed him may appoint another surveyor in his place.

The wording '*may* appoint another surveyor in his place' appears to suggest that in those particular and unusual circumstances the appointment of a surveyor could be arbitrary or optional but this is not the case as compliance with the provisions of the statute obliges the parties to make the appointment if matters are disputed.

Should matters have developed as far as the selection of the third surveyor then, in the unfortunate event of the death of an appointed surveyor, or should he become unable to act, the need to appoint another surveyor in his place may be obviated by the remaining surveyor calling in the third surveyor to join with him in signing the award – see Section 10(10).

Problems can arise where an appointed surveyor's personal situation alters or becomes different from that which prevailed at the time he had accepted his appointment to act; he could suffer a physical injury or become ill; or he could, through circumstances beyond his control, find that his qualifying status as defined under Section 20 had changed so as to make him party to the dispute and result in his having a conflict of interest; or he might emigrate or move house such that distance from the site of the matters in dispute would prohibit him from continuing in his appointment.

Any of the above suggested, but by no means exhaustive, list of examples can be considered as a legitimate reason for an appointed surveyor to become incapable or deem himself incapable of acting. However, it is unacceptable for a surveyor to deem himself incapable of acting if the relevant conditions applying at the time he accepted his appointment have not altered in any way capable of justifying such action.

Section 10(6)(a), (b) and (7)(a), (b)

(6) If a surveyor–

(a) appointed under paragraph (b) of subsection (1) by a party to the dispute; or

(b) appointed under subsection (4) or (5),

refuses to act effectively, the surveyor of the other party may proceed to act *ex parte* and anything so done by him shall be as effectual as if he had been an agreed surveyor.

(7) If a surveyor–

(a) appointed under paragraph (b) of subsection (1) by a party to the dispute; or

(b) appointed under subsection (4) or (5),

neglects to act effectively for a period of ten days beginning with the day on which either party or the surveyor of the other party serves a request on him, the surveyor of the other party may proceed to act *ex parte* in respect of the subject matter of the request and anything so done by him shall be as effectual as if he had been an agreed surveyor.

A surveyor has a duty to properly perform the functions for which he is appointed under statute and is obliged to comply with the provisions of the Act to effectively resolve the dispute between the parties.

If it becomes evident that an appointed surveyor refuses to act effectively by not complying with the provisions of the Act and, by his refusal or inaction, prejudices or hinders in some way the resolution process, the surveyor appointed by the other party may proceed to act *ex parte* on his own or separately.

Should a surveyor proceed to act *ex parte* he is then entitled to determine the disputed matters and to make such awards as are necessary with the same authority as he would have were he to have been appointed as an agreed surveyor.

Section 10(6) is concerned with the refusal to act effectively, and a consequence of this refusal could be to allow the other surveyor to proceed on his own and perhaps complete the resolution of the disputed matters by making what in effect would be an agreed surveyor's award.

A surveyor would only be justified in choosing to take the extreme option of proceeding *ex parte* on the basis that the other surveyor had, in some intentional way, expressly refused to do something as specific as, for example, signing an award, or had refused to consider taking any further action to determine the disputed matters or until such time as his fee had been agreed.

An award made *ex parte* will most probably be subject to challenge on appeal by whichever of the parties to the dispute considers that they have been unfairly treated consequent to a surveyor taking such peremptory action.

It is more usual for a situation to arise where a surveyor neglects to act rather than refuses to act effectively, and in that instance either of the parties to the dispute or a surveyor to one of the parties can serve on the other surveyor a written request that he takes some specific action to progress matters. If no effective action is taken within ten days of the receipt of the request, the requesting party's surveyor can then proceed to act *ex parte* in respect of the subject matter of the request.

Therefore to this extent a surveyor will be at risk of being superseded by the other surveyor only in respect of the matter in which he has defaulted. He might not have taken some necessary definite action or actions which, among others, could include material delay in answering correspondence, failing to make a required statutory appointment, failing to agree the selection of a third surveyor or failing to take some other specific and required step – see Section 10(4)(b).

Section 10(8)(a), (b)

(8) If either surveyor appointed under subsection (1)(b) by a party to the dispute refuses to select a third surveyor under subsection (1) or (9), or neglects to do so for a period of ten days beginning with the day on which the other surveyor serves a request on him–

    (a) the appointing officer; or

    (b) in cases where the relevant appointing officer or his employer is a party to the dispute, the Secretary of State,

may on the application of either surveyor select a third surveyor who shall have the same power and authority as if he had been selected under subsection (1) or subsection (9).

This subsection concerns the selection of a third surveyor when, in the first instance, either of the two appointed surveyors refuses or neglects to make the required selection and, in the second instance, where the local authority itself is a party to the dispute.

Should an appointed surveyor refuse to agree the selection of a third surveyor and, after the elapse of ten days from his receipt of a request from the other surveyor, neglect to make the selection, either surveyor may make application for the selection to the appointing officer of the building control section of the local authority which administers the area where the works are to be carried out.

If his selection is made by the appointing officer of the local authority the third surveyor will have the same power and authority to act as if he had been selected by the appointed surveyors under the provisions of Section 10(1) or Section 10(9).

An application to a local authority's appointing officer may be considered much in the same way as an application to the local authority for planning or building regulations consent and as such the application may incur local authority charges. An ensuing award should cite the particular reasons necessitating the selection of the third surveyor by the appointing officer and, if appropriate, award any incurred costs to be paid by the owner whose appointed surveyor had refused to make the selection.

Following the refusal or neglect by either surveyor to select a third surveyor where the local authority or its employee, the relevant appointing officer, is a party to the dispute, either surveyor may apply to the Secretary of State to make the selection.

A third surveyor selected by the Secretary of State will have the same power and authority to act as if he had been selected by the two appointed surveyors under the provisions of Section 10(1) or Section 10(9).

Section 10(9)(a)–(c)

(9) If a third surveyor selected under subsection (1)(b)–

    (a) refuses to act;

    (b) neglects to act for a period of ten days beginning with the day on which either party or the surveyor appointed by either party serves a request on him; or

    (c) dies, or becomes or deems himself incapable of acting, before the dispute is settled,

the other two of the three surveyors shall forthwith select another surveyor in his place with the same power and authority.

If for any reason the selected third surveyor refuses to act or neglects to act after ten days of having been served a written request to act by either of the parties to the dispute or by either of their appointed surveyors or if he dies or becomes, or deems himself, incapable of acting then the other two appointed surveyors must immediately select another third surveyor in his place and their selection will have the same power and authority as did the previously selected third surveyor.

Section 10(10)(a), (b)

(10) The agreed surveyor or as the case may be the three surveyors or any two of them shall settle by award any matter–

    (a) which is connected with any work to which this Act relates, and

    (b) which is in dispute between the building owner and the adjoining owner.

An adjoining owner's written dissent to a written notice served on him by a building owner gives rise to a dispute between the owners, and then matters must be settled either by the agreed surveyor or by the two appointed surveyors or, infrequently, by one of the appointed surveyors in conjunction with the agreed surveyor when one of the two appointed surveyors may be in the wrong or in disagreement with the other surveyor. It would be extremely unusual for all three surveyors to have to combine to settle the matters in dispute.

Although the Act refers to settling by award any matter which is connected with any work to which the Act relates, this reference cannot include work which had already been started, even completed, without the mandatory service of notice.

Any attempt to rectify a situation where work had been unlawfully proceeded with would require the willingness of both parties to accept and agree that the building owner serves on the adjoining owner appropriate written notice and to which the adjoining owner will formally dissent. The consequential appointment of surveyors should regularise compliance with the legal process necessary to resolve the disputed matters.

Section 10(11)

> (11) Either of the parties or either of the surveyors appointed by the parties may call upon the third surveyor selected in pursuance of this section to determine the disputed matters and he shall make the necessary award.

Either party to the dispute or either of their appointed surveyors is entitled to call in the third surveyor when the two appointed surveyors are unable themselves to resolve their differences.

Usually it is for one of the two appointed surveyors to call in the third surveyor to independently determine the issues on which they disagree, and although a party to the dispute is prohibited from dismissing his appointed surveyor or influencing his actions, he is allowed to disagree with that surveyor's opinion and might himself prefer to ask the third surveyor to award on the disputed matters.

Apart from probable delays to the progress of the work, calling in the third surveyor will inevitably result in a liability for costs for one or other of the parties in dispute, and it is advisable that an appointed surveyor makes the party that appointed him fully aware of this potential liability.

Section 10(12)(a)–(c)

> (12) An award may determine–
>
> (a) the right to execute any work;
>
> (b) the time and manner of executing any work; and
>
> (c) any other matter arising out of or incidental to the dispute including the costs of making the award;
>
> but any period appointed by the award for executing any work shall not unless otherwise agreed between the building owner and the adjoining owner begin to run until after the expiration of the period prescribed by this Act for service of the notice in respect of which the dispute arises or is deemed to have arisen.

The words of this subsection are illustrative of the wide jurisdiction given to the appointed surveyors to enable them to deal with matters not only directly relating to the resolution of disputes concerned with the notifiable work itself but also to extend this jurisdiction to determine issues ancillary and additional to the dispute.

The Act empowers the appointed surveyors to determine the fundamentals relating to the right to carry out work, including its scope and extent, and to deal with matters as diverse as deciding when and in what manner authorised work may be undertaken. They may rule on the liability for costs and expenses, and perhaps payment of compensation, but they may only determine and award on matters covered by the Act. An award will be considered invalid if it decides on matters of common law or is perhaps made consequent to service of an invalid notice and it is similarly invalid if it purports to retrospectively resolve disputes arising from work which had been unlawfully started before notice had been given.

Although an award cannot authorise any notifiable work started before service of formal notice it can provide for the resolution of matters incidental to but not necessarily those that were cited in the subject matter of a notice.

It is often the situation that prior to the service of notice, dissent to which initiates his consequent appointment, a surveyor will advise on the relevance of the Act in relation to a building owner's proposals and, as his agent, will serve an appropriate notice on the building owner's behalf.

It is often suggested that surveyors have no jurisdiction to determine and award on issues that might arise before service of notice but it is appropriate that an account for fees incurred in giving advice to his client or an account for costs engendered by related correspondence or documentation leading to the necessary production and service of notices could properly be considered as incidental to the dispute and so be legitimately awarded.

The Act provides for a period of time to run between the date of service of notice and the date on which the notified work may start: work subject to the provisions of Section 1 and Section 6 requires a period of one calendar month, work subject to the provisions of Section 2 requires a period of two months. The date on which building owner proposes to start the work should be stated on the notice and it must be in accordance with the provisions of the Act, and unless the parties to the dispute agree to an earlier date, work may not commence until the appropriate time has run.

There is no requirement to agree a limit to the period of time needed by the building owner for starting and completing the authorised work nor is it required that the adjoining owner be notified of its completion. Should the surveyors consider that it would better serve the parties' interests if the work were to be subject to a time limit, they can award to this effect; disagreement between the surveyors on this point could be resolved by a third surveyor's award which, as for all awards, is also subject to appeal.

Section 10(13)(a)–(c)

(13) The reasonable costs incurred in–

    (a) making or obtaining an award under this section;

    (b) reasonable inspections of work to which the award relates; and

    (c) any other matter arising out of the dispute,

shall be paid by such of the parties as the surveyor or surveyors making the award determine.

The appointed surveyors are empowered to decide on any of the issues relating to liability for costs incurred not only in making or obtaining an award or for making reasonable inspections of the work to which the Act relates but also for costs incurred in resolving the issues and awarding on any other matter arising out of the dispute.

The building owner will always be responsible for the outcome of the procedures started with his notice of intended work and is normally responsible for the surveyor's fees and for other costs including those incurred by consultants giving specialist advice or services. Specialist advice in this context might be that sought from a structural engineer who would be asked by an adjoining owner's surveyor to comment on the engineering aspects of the building owner's proposals; it should be remembered that the structural engineer or other consultant, perhaps an advising solicitor, has neither a remit, an appointment nor a nomination to act in the procedures leading to an award and can only give advice to an appointed surveyor sufficient to assist him in determining the issues in dispute.

Engineering advice is sometimes called for but it should only take the form of a general appraisal of the building owner's proposals; there is no requirement for a detailed and exhaustive check of the building owner's engineer's designs and calculations nor is it appropriate to propose alternative designs for reasons of preference.

In certain circumstances an engineer might be asked to make site inspections to check that the work on which he is advising is being carried out in accordance with the terms of the award.

An advising engineer, solicitor or other consultant is generally not named in an award, and fees and expenses incurred for his contribution to the resolution of the disputed matters are considered to be disbursements payable by the surveyor who has sought the consultant's advice and with whom he is technically in contract. Disbursements should be identified as such and included as a part of a surveyor's awarded fee.

When the level of fees or disbursements claimed by an adjoining owner's surveyor is the subject of disagreement between the surveyors the matter can be referred to the third surveyor for his determination and award but it should be remembered that the third surveyor's award will also contain directions as to the payment of his own fee. If the award determines that the adjoining owner's surveyor's claim is excessive it will direct that the third surveyor's fee be paid by the adjoining owner; before the matter is referred, the adjoining owner's surveyor should make the adjoining owner fully aware of this possibility.

A building owner who might disagree with the terms of an award can appeal it under the provisions of Section 10(17) if he considers that its provisions are unjust or that the fees that surveyors have awarded are excessive or misdirected.

Section 10(14)

> Where the surveyors appointed by the parties make an award the surveyors shall serve it forthwith on the parties.

Having made an award, the appointed surveyors have a duty to serve it without delay on the parties in dispute. Although it is customary for a surveyor to serve the award on the party who appointed him, either surveyor can serve the award on either or both of the parties if, due to prevailing circumstances, that is what is expedient.

Section 10(15)(a), (b)

> (15) Where an award is made by the third surveyor–
>
>   (a) he shall, after payment of the costs of the award, serve it forthwith on the parties or their appointed surveyors; and
>
>   (b) if it is served on their appointed surveyors, they shall serve it forthwith on the parties.

Having stated his fee incurred in making his award, and having announced that the award is ready for service, the third surveyor must serve it directly on the parties or their appointed surveyors as soon as his fee is paid. If the award is sent to the surveyors they must immediately serve it on the parties.

A party wanting to lose no time in obtaining the award might opt to pay the third surveyor's fee but, without prior knowledge of the contents of the award, may find that the responsibility for payment has been awarded against the other party and will seek to be reimbursed by him.

Section 10(16)

> The award shall be conclusive and shall not except as provided by this section be questioned in any court.

An award made by appointed surveyors is conclusive on their signature, and the Act makes no provision for it to be questioned or to become the object of controversy other than to provide that it may be subject to appeal.

That an award may be considered conclusive will not in itself protect a building owner from the consequences of his actions when his responsibility to an adjoining owner or to third parties extends his liability for latent damage or damage directly or incidentally caused by his authorised work.

Section 10(17)(a), (b)

(17) Either of the parties to the dispute may, within the period of fourteen days beginning with the day on which an award made under this section is served on him, appeal to the county court against the award and the county court may–

(a) rescind the award or modify it in such manner as the court thinks fit; and

(b) make such order as to costs as the court thinks fit.

The parties in dispute have a right to appeal an award within 14 days from the date of their receipt of its service and it is customary for the appointed surveyors to provide information to that effect in the award itself as well as in correspondence covering its service.

Either of the parties to the dispute may appeal to the county court on any aspect of the subject matter of an award or on the validity of the award itself, and the court can modify the award in any way it thinks fit or, if it is considered appropriate, rescind it.

The court can make orders concerning any continuing liability or responsibility for payment of costs and give directions as to payment.

An appointed surveyor, independent of the owners and excluded from being a party to the dispute (see Section 20), is not himself entitled to any rights of appeal even though he may be directly affected by the scope of the courts' jurisdiction which can decide on a wide range of matters including, for example, those concerning the legitimacy of his own appointment or the payment of his fees.

Section 11 Expenses

Section 11(1), (2)

(1) Except as provided under this section expenses of work under this Act shall be defrayed by the building owner.

(2) Any dispute as to responsibility for expenses shall be settled as provided in section 10.

The Act says that, other than for certain particular instances described later in this section, the building owner shall defray the expenses for any authorised work he carries out.

More specifically, where an adjoining owner does not agree to the building of a party wall or a party fence wall on the line of junction, a building owner is directly responsible for the expenses arising from building the new wall entirely on his own land (Section 1(4)), or where he builds a wall at the line of junction on his own land but places its foundations on the adjoining owner's land – Section 1(7).

He is also liable for expenses incurred when, in carrying out his authorised work, he safeguards or underpins or is required to underpin the foundations of an adjoining owner's building or structure – Section 6(3).

The question also arises as to an adjoining owner's liability for any contribution to expenses he might have to make in recognition of the benefit that may, for example, accrue to the stability of his building being enhanced by the building owner's work.

Section 11(3)

An expense mentioned in section 1(3)(b) shall be defrayed as there mentioned.

An agreement for a party wall or party fence wall to be built on the line of junction will generally provide that payment of the consequent expenses is apportioned in accordance with each party's individual and particular use of the wall at the time it is built. An example might be when the major portion of the expenses are borne by a building owner when the party wall forms an external wall of his building but acts only as a boundary wall to the adjoining owner's land.

If an adjoining owner makes any subsequent use of the party wall, he is obliged to pay such expenses as would have been incurred in its construction at the rates which prevail at the time his use is made of it and not at the rates which applied when it was originally built – Section 11(11).

Section 11(4)(a), (b)

(4) Where work is carried out in exercise of the right mentioned in section 2(2)(a), and the work is necessary on account of defect or want of repair of the structure or wall concerned, the expenses shall be defrayed by the building owner and the adjoining owner in such proportion as has regard to–

    (a) the use which the owners respectively make or may make of the structure or wall concerned; and

    (b) responsibility for the defect or want of repair concerned, if more than one owner makes use of the structure or wall concerned.

Where wants of repair, or the remedy of defects in a party wall, party fence wall or an external wall belonging to a building owner and abutting a party structure or party fence wall, require that it is underpinned, thickened or raised in accordance with the rights granted in Section 2(2)(a) the expenses incurred are to be defrayed in proportion to the use each owner makes of the wall.

The building owner will be solely responsible for the cost of new work carried out for his own benefit, but he is entitled to recoup a proportion of that expenditure from an adjoining owner or owners when the use they make or may make of the wall contributes to its defect or wants of repair.

Section 11(4)(a) says 'the use which the owners respectively make or may make of the structure or wall concerned' which clearly indicates that not only is an adjoining owner's past use of the wall considered to be relevant in assessing his legal liability for payment of expenses but also that the liability increases if his anticipated future use of the wall or structure dictates that greater and more expensive remedial works might need to be undertaken.

Section 11(4)(b) says 'responsibility for the defect or want of repair concerned, if more than one owner makes use of the structure or wall concerned.' The reference here is to defects or wants of repair caused by a past use made of the wall or structure by an adjoining owner or owners and to the degree of responsibility each owner has in contributing to the situation that gave rise to the damage or defect.

Section 11(5)(a), (b)

(5) Where work is carried out in exercise of the right mentioned in section 2(2)(b) the expenses shall be defrayed by the building owner and the adjoining owner in such proportion as has regard to–

(a) the use which the owners respectively make or may make of the structure or wall concerned; and

(b) responsibility for the defect or want of repair concerned, if more than one owner makes use of the structure or wall concerned.

Where a defect or want of repair requires the making good, repairing or demolishing and rebuilding of a party structure or party fence wall (as in Section 2(2)(b)) costs will be apportioned as for Section 11(4).

While an owner's liability to pay a proportion of the cost of necessary repairs is directly related to the use he makes of the wall or structure, it can, for example, also extend to include damage to its foundations due to fractures in his drains or by desiccation caused by tree roots from his next door garden. If there are several owners involved, the liability for costs to make good damage and remedy defects should be in direct proportion to the contribution to the cause of the damage made by each individual owner.

Section 11(6)

(6) Where the adjoining premises are laid open in exercise of the right mentioned in section 2(2)(e) a fair allowance in respect of disturbance and inconvenience shall be paid by the building owner to the adjoining owner or occupier.

When exercising the right conferred by Section 2(2)(e), a building owner may demolish a party structure, lay open an adjoining owner's premises and rebuild to his new requirements an existing party structure which is of insufficient height or strength or is inadequate for his intended purposes, and he has to pay an adjoining owner or occupier a fair allowance for any disturbance and inconvenience the work causes. It has previously been suggested in Section 7(3) that the extreme and drastic action of laying open adjoining premises should be the option of last resort. It should also be noted that the sum to be considered as a fair allowance should be agreed between the parties prior to the commencement of the work and not assessed as compensation for any loss later incurred.

Section 11(7)(a), (b)

(7) Where a building owner proposes to reduce the height of a party wall or party fence wall under section 2(2)(m) the adjoining owner may serve a counter notice under section 4 requiring the building owner to maintain the existing height of the wall, and in such case the adjoining owner shall pay to the building owner a due proportion of the cost of the wall so far as it exceeds–

   (a) two metres in height; or

   (b) the height currently enclosed upon by the building of the adjoining owner.

When an adjoining owner uses a party wall or party fence wall solely as a boundary wall to his premises, a building owner may demolish and rebuild it or reduce its height to a minimum of two metres. If an adjoining owner wishes to maintain the wall at a height greater than two metres, he must serve on the building owner a counter notice to that effect and must pay the building owner a proportion of the cost involved in maintaining that part of the wall where its height exceeds two metres.

If a party wall forms an enclosing wall to an adjoining owner's building, a building owner may not reduce its height to a level less than that currently required by the adjoining owner to maintain the enclosure of his building. If the adjoining owner requires the wall to have a parapet, or if a parapet is needed to satisfy building regulations, it may be left in situ above the enclosing wall at no cost to the adjoining owner.

Section 11(8)

(8) Where the building owner is required to make good damage under this Act the adjoining owner has a right to require that the expenses of such making good be determined in accordance with section 10 and paid to him in lieu of the carrying out of work to make the damage good.

While the Act requires that a building owner must compensate an adjoining owner or occupier for any loss or damage that he causes in carrying out his authorised work, it also provides that the adjoining owner or occupier is entitled to opt for an agreed payment to be made in lieu of the repairs being carried out by the building owner.

The Act specifically obliges the building owner only to make good or repair damage caused by work carried out under:

Section 2(2)(a), underpinning, thickening or raising a party structure, party fence wall or a building owner's external wall built against a party structure or party fence wall.

Section 2(2)(e), demolition and rebuilding of a party structure.

Section 2(2)(f), cutting into a party structure for any purpose.

Section 2(2)(j), cutting into an adjoining owner's building to insert a flashing.

If the adjoining owner requires payment in lieu of the building owner carrying out the repair works, and if a disagreement arises as to the extent or cost of the damage to be rectified or to its implementation, the matter must be referred to the surveyors in accordance with the provisions of Section 10.

Section 11(9)(a), (b)

(9) Where–

    (a) works are carried out, and

    (b) some of the works are carried out at the request of the adjoining owner or in pursuance of a requirement made by him,

he shall defray the expenses of carrying out the works requested or required by him.

With the exception of the costs arising from safeguarding or underpinning the foundations of his building (Section 6(3)), such costs being payable by the building owner, the adjoining owner is responsible for the cost of any work he has requested or required of the building owner having served him a counter notice under Section 4.

Section 11(10)(a), (b)

(11) Where–

    (a) consent in writing has been given to the construction of special foundations on land of an adjoining owner; and

    (b) the adjoining owner erects any building or structure and its cost is found to be increased by reason of the existence of the said foundations,

the owner of the building to which the said foundations belong shall, on receiving an account with any necessary invoices and other supporting documents within the period of two months beginning with the day of the completion of the work by the adjoining owner, repay to the adjoining owner so much of the cost as is due to the existence of the said foundations.

Whereas Section 1(6) permits simple mass concrete foundations to be placed on an adjoining owner's land, a building owner may not place reinforced concrete or concrete encased steel foundations on that land without the adjoining owner's written consent.

If the adjoining owner wishes to erect a building or structure on his own land, and the cost of its construction is increased as a consequence of the existence of special foundations, he is entitled to recoup the amount of the increase from the building owner.

An incumbent owner of special foundations may be unaware of them and may not be the original owner who obtained written consent for them to be placed on the adjoining land, and it may be that the incumbent adjoining owner is not the original adjoining owner who gave written consent to allow them, but the passage of time will not relieve the owner of the special foundations of his obligation to pay compensation to his neighbour for the increased construction costs arising from their existence.

Section 11(11)

(11) Where use is subsequently made by the adjoining owner of work carried out solely at the expense of the building owner the adjoining owner shall pay a due proportion of the expenses incurred by the building owner in carrying out that work; and for this purpose he shall be taken to have incurred expenses calculated by reference to what the cost of the work would be if it were carried out at the time when that subsequent use is made.

When a building owner builds a party wall on the line of junction it becomes in joint ownership, but if at the time it is built no contribution to the cost of its construction nor use of it is made by the adjoining owner it is the building owner only who will bear the cost of building it.

If at some subsequent date the adjoining owner, or his heirs, want to make use of the wall or a part of it, they must pay to the building owner, or his heirs, a due proportion of the expenses incurred, not at the time the wall was built but calculated to be the costs prevailing at the time he makes use of it.

It is important to recognise the difference in context between ownership and use, and where one party might own the wall and the other party may benefit by making use of it. This can happen without the adjoining owner having to carry out any otherwise necessary construction works or committing trespass.

An illustration of this might be where the building owner, at his own expense, raises a party wall to a level substantially higher than the level of the adjoining owner's flat roof. The wall abuts and encloses one side of the flat roof which, after the party wall has been raised, the adjoining owner proposes to use as a terrace. On the party wall side of the flat roof terrace, the regulation for a necessary guard rail will be satisfied by a 1.1 m high section of the party wall. The building owner is then entitled to ask the adjoining owner to reimburse him a proportion of the cost of building a 1.1 m high section of the party wall in lieu of the adjoining owner having to provide for himself the regulation guard rail.

Architects making applications for planning permission should be aware of the anomalous situation concerning 'ownership' of a party wall when compliance with the planning Acts requires one of the alternative declarations to be made in Certificate 'A', the standard form printed here.

**TOWN & COUNTRY PLANNING
(GENERAL DEVELOPMENT PROCEDURE) ORDER 1995**

CERTIFICATE UNDER ARTICLE 7

CERTIFICATE A (a)

I certify that:

On the day 21 days before the date of the accompanying application/appeal* nobody, except the applicant/appellant, was the owner (b) of any part of the land to which the application/appeal* relates.

Signed...............................

* On behalf of ....

Date.................................

* Delete where appropriate

Typically, the boundary line or line of junction will most probably be centrally placed in the thickness of the party wall and, for the purposes of a planning application, will denote the legal limit of the curtilage of the applicant's land.

The raising of the whole of the party wall will be necessary when, for example, the development of the roof space of a terraced house includes a dormer. However, while this is permitted under the Party Wall etc. Act 1996, it also involves the building owner in raising a wall half of which is within the curtilage of his land and half of which belongs to the adjoining owner.

It is apparent that, as an alternative, the completion of Certificate 'B' could suggest, wrongly, that an adjoining owner has the potential to object to a right conferred on a building owner under Section 2(2)(a), that is to say 'ownership' taking precedence over 'use'.

Section 12 Security for expenses

Section 12(1)

> (1) An adjoining owner may serve a notice requiring the building owner before he begins any work in the exercise of the rights conferred by this Act to give such security as may be agreed between the owners or in the event of dispute determined in accordance with section 10.

In specific circumstances, Section 12 of the Act gives both the building owner and the adjoining owner the right to demand, one from the other, security for expenses arising from default; from the building owner in relation to the execution of authorised work and from the adjoining owner in relation to work under Section 4(1) carried out on his behalf by the building owner.

Having given an adjoining owner due notice, a building owner may exercise his right to proceed with authorised work which, in all required aspects, complies with the Act but there is no provision for him to give the adjoining owner evidence of his financial status or even of his solvency before he starts the work.

Without the building owner being required to deposit some agreed amount of money as security against possible future claims, an adjoining owner might, for any reason, find himself having to pay to repair or reconstruct his property should the building owner not complete the authorised work or perhaps fail to pay sums that have been awarded or calculated as compensation under Section 7, or monies to which an adjoining owner is entitled under Section 1(7) or Section 11(6).

The adjoining owner's right to security must be exercised before the authorised work is started, and the procedure is initiated by a notice requiring that sufficient and adequate funds are to be secured against the possibility of default by the building owner. The notice is served on him by the adjoining owner or, if the adjoining owner gives him authority, by the adjoining owner's surveyor.

If the owners disagree as to whether security needs to be provided, or as to its amount, the appointed surveyors will determine the issues in accordance with Section 10. It is important to note that even though the adjoining owner might have given his written consent to the building owner's proposed work and as a consequence the appointment of surveyors was not required, the need to resolve the dispute over security would itself necessitate their appointment.

Section 12(2)(a), (b)

(2) Where–

(a) in the exercise of the rights conferred by this Act an adjoining owner requires the building owner to carry out any work the expenses of which are to be defrayed in whole or in part by the adjoining owner; or

(b) an adjoining owner serves a notice on the building owner under subsection (1),

the building owner may before beginning the work to which the requirement or notice relates serve a notice on the adjoining owner requiring him to give such security as may be agreed between the owners or in the event of dispute determined in accordance with section 10.

A similar right to security for expenses is available to the building owner from the adjoining owner but the circumstances regulating the procedures are rather different. As before, and consequent on the service of notice, disagreement between the owners on the need for such security or disagreement as to its amount or to any other of its aspects the matter must be determined under the provisions of Section 10.

It is obvious that when work is carried out by a building owner on behalf of an adjoining owner it needs to be paid for. The building owner is entitled to serve notice on the adjoining owner for security for expenses to provide against the possibility of the adjoining owner refusing to pay for his requested work or in some other way defaulting on his obligations. It is interesting to note that the Act gives a building owner the right to demand this security from the adjoining owner not only as a consequence of being asked to carry out the adjoining owner's work but also, and almost punitively, as a quid pro quo reciprocation of the adjoining owner's right to request that security for expenses be provided to him.

Section 12(3)(a), (b)

(3) If within the period of one month beginning with–

(a) the day on which a notice is served under subsection (2); or

(b) in the event of dispute, the date of the determination by the surveyor or surveyors,

the adjoining owner does not comply with the notice or the determination, the requirement or notice by him to which the building owner's notice under that subsection relates shall cease to have effect.

A building owner should not be unnecessarily delayed in carrying out his authorised work, and while it is required that an adjoining owner must serve a security notice before the building owner's work is started, no time limits apply to the building owner's response, nor must he comply with an award for security made against him. It is tacit that a building owner ignoring the provisions of Section 12(1) runs the risk of being restrained by the courts if work is started before he gives the required security.

No such latitude is available to an adjoining owner, and this subsection deals with the procedure governing the short time limits allowed for him to respond to a security notice served on him by the building owner.

If within a month, beginning with the day an adjoining owner is served a security notice, he does not properly respond to the building owner's request for security relating to the adjoining owner's request made under Section 12(2) or, in the event of a dispute, by a date determined by an award, the adjoining owner's request to the building owner will cease to have effect, and the building owner will be released from his obligation to carry out the adjoining owner's requested work.

Ideally, the security should be provided in the form of an agreed sum of money assessed in proportion to the risk to be covered, deposited in an escrow account opened in the names of the three surveyors and released under their joint signatures only when all and any claims against it have been satisfied. This option of providing security has the obvious advantage that the matters will be under the control of surveyors appointed under statute and who are not parties to the dispute that gives rise to the need for the security and who are competent to assess the validity of a claim made against it.

Alternative options for effecting security might include those providing security bonds or collateral warranties, or they might be for the security given by a third party or a parent company guarantee, but these options inevitably delay the resolution and processing of claims.

Section 13 Account for work carried out

Section 13(1)(a), (b)

(1) Within the period of two months beginning with the day of the completion of any work executed by a building owner of which the expenses are to be wholly or partially defrayed by an adjoining owner in accordance with section 11 the building owner shall serve on the adjoining owner an account in writing showing–

(a) particulars and expenses of the work; and

(b) any deductions to which the adjoining owner or any other person is entitled in respect of old materials or otherwise;

and in preparing the account the work shall be estimated and valued at fair average rates and prices according to the nature of the work, the locality and the cost of labour and materials prevailing at the time when the work is executed.

Where an adjoining owner is required to contribute to the building owner's expenses in accordance with the provisions of Section 11 he must be served a written statement of account giving detailed evidence of his liability to the building owner.

The building owner must serve the account within two months beginning with the day that he completes the work, and its compilation is required to demonstrate the fair and average rates and prices for labour and materials applying at the time the work was undertaken. It should clearly indicate any allowance made for the use of second-hand materials, or materials or services provided by the adjoining owner, and any costs that could have been influenced by the specific nature of the work or by it having to have been executed in a particular geographical location.

If after the expiration of two months from the completion of the work no account has been served on the adjoining owner, the building owner loses his right to claim.

Section 13(2), (3)

(2) Within the period of one month beginning with the day of service of the said account the adjoining owner may serve on the building owner a notice stating any objection he may have thereto and thereupon a dispute shall be deemed to have arisen between the parties.

(3) If within that period of one month the adjoining owner does not serve notice under subsection (2) he shall be deemed to have no objection to the account.

Having been served an account by the building owner, the adjoining owner has one month from the date of its service to object to it by serving a counter notice on the building owner. The adjoining owner's notice must state the reasons for his objections, and its service on the building owner gives rise to the occurrence of a deemed dispute; matters must be resolved under the provisions of Section 10.

If within a period of one month from the date of service of the building owner's account, the adjoining owner serves no counter notice, makes no written objection to it or is silent on the matter, he is deemed to have accepted it and accordingly should make due payment to the building owner. In default, the recovery of the debt may be dealt with by application to the magistrates' court in accordance with the provisions of Section 17.

Section 14 Settlement of account

Section 14(1), (2)

(1) All expenses to be defrayed by an adjoining owner in accordance with an account served under section 13 shall be paid by the adjoining owner.

(2) Until an adjoining owner pays to the building owner such expenses as aforesaid the property in any works executed under this Act to which the expenses relate shall be vested solely in the building owner.

The adjoining owner must make payment of an account served on him under Section 13 and to which he has made no objection. Until he makes due payment for the work carried out on his behalf, the work will remain in the sole ownership of the building owner.

It is difficult to understand the value to a building owner of becoming the sole owner of, say, a party wall or party fence wall only as a result of the adjoining owner's default, and the building owner is owed the due proportion of the cost of the work he has carried out on behalf of the adjoining owner (Section 1). While the adjoining owner's debt remains unpaid the building owner is the legal owner of the whole of the wall founded on the land of both owners, and any use made of it by the adjoining owner will constitute trespass.

Section 15 Service of notices etc.

Section 15(1)(a)–(c)

(1) A notice or other document required or authorised to be served under this Act may be served on a person–

(a) by delivering it to him in person;

(b) by sending it by post to him at his usual or last-known residence or place of business in the United Kingdom; or

(c) in the case of a body corporate, by delivering it to the secretary or clerk of the body corporate at its registered or principal office or sending it by post to the secretary or clerk of that body corporate at that office.

The Act is specific in its requirements that regulate the manner in which authorised service of notices and documents have to be served on persons or corporate bodies.

When notice is to be served on an individual and the option of personal service is unavailable then service by post is advocated. The documents should be sent to the person at his usual or last known residential address or at his place of business in the United Kingdom. A notice will be invalid if it is served on a person having his usual residential or business address outside the United Kingdom.

If notice is to be served on a body corporate it should be delivered to the secretary or clerk of the company at its registered or principal office or by sending it by post to him at that office, wherever it is situated.

Section 15(2)(a), (b)

(2) In the case of a notice or other document required or authorised to be served under this Act on a person as owner of premises, it may alternatively be served by–

(a) addressing it "the owner" of the premises (naming them); and

(b) delivering it to a person on the premises or, if no person to whom it can be delivered is found there, fixing it to a conspicuous part of the premises.

It is often the case that notices or documents need to be served at premises where the name of the owner of the premises is not known.

The notice or document should be addressed to 'the owner' of the premises, giving its address, and personally delivered to someone on the premises. If no one is there to accept service of the notice, it may be fixed to a part of the premises, usually the front door, where it can easily be seen.

The time for a response to a notice runs from the day it is served, and if the proposal is to fix it to the premises, it is prudent to have the procedure witnessed, photographed or otherwise verified.

Section 16 Offences

Section 16(1)(a), (b)

(1) If–

(a) an occupier of land or premises refuses to permit a person to do anything which he is entitled to do with regard to the land or premises under section 8(1) or (5); and

(b) the occupier knows or has reasonable cause to believe that the person is so entitled,

the occupier is guilty of an offence.

An occupier may be neither an adjoining owner nor someone who is aware of the dispute, but it is an offence for the occupier of land or premises to refuse to permit someone to enter or carry out work on those premises under the provisions of Section 8(1) or (5) when the occupier knows or has reasonable cause to believe that the person wishing to carry out the work is so entitled.

Section 16(2)(a), (b)

(2) If–

    (a) a person hinders or obstructs a person in attempting to do anything which he is entitled to do with regard to land or premises under section 8(1) or (5); and

    (b) the first-mentioned person knows or has reasonable cause to believe that the other person is so entitled,

the first-mentioned person is guilty of an offence.

If someone being on land or premises in accordance with Section 8(1) or (5) for the purpose of carrying out work, making inspections or for any other purpose in relation to the dispute is hindered or obstructed by an occupier who knows, or has reasonable cause to believe, that the person is entitled to be on the premises the person causing the obstruction is guilty of an offence.

Section 16(3)

(3) A person guilty of an offence under subsection (1) or (2) is liable on summary conviction to a fine of an amount not exceeding level 3 on the standard scale.

Someone guilty of an offence under Section 16(1) or (2) is, on summary conviction in the magistrates' court, liable to a fine of an amount not exceeding level 3 on the standard scale fixed by the Criminal Justice Act 1982 as amended by the relevant section of the Criminal Justice Act 1991.

Section 17 Recovery of sums

Any sum payable in pursuance of this Act (otherwise than by way of fine) shall be recoverable summarily as a civil debt.

In situations where an owner fails to make payment to which the other owner is entitled under an award or, pursuant to Section 12(1), by agreement between the owners, the matter is referred to the magistrates' court and, on the provision of evidence – perhaps the award itself – the sum owed is recoverable summarily as a civil debt.

Section 18 Exception in case of Temples etc.

Section 18(1)(a)–(d) and (2)

(1) This Act shall not apply to land which is situated in inner London and in which there is an interest belonging to–

(a) the Honourable Society of the Inner Temple,

(b) the Honourable Society of the Middle Temple,

(c) the Honourable Society of Lincoln's Inn, or

(d) the Honourable Society of Gray's Inn.

(2) The reference in subsection (1) to inner London is to Greater London other than the outer London boroughs.

This section cites the properties owned by the Inns of Court which, by being situated in the inner London boroughs of Greater London, are exempt from the provisions of the Act. However, pursuant to the Act, notice may be served on the owners of those properties when they are adjoining owners.

The exemption does not apply to properties owned by the Inns of Court and which are situated outside Greater London.

Section 19 The Crown

Section 19(1)(a)–(c) and (2)(a), (b)

(1) This Act shall apply to land in which there is–

(a) an interest belonging to Her Majesty in right of the Crown,

(b) an interest belonging to a government department, or

(c) an interest held in trust for Her Majesty for the purposes of any such department.

(2) This Act shall apply to–

(a) land which is vested in, but not occupied by, Her Majesty in right of the Duchy of Lancaster;

(b) land which is vested in, but not occupied by, the possessor for the time being of the Duchy of Cornwall.

Crown properties are not exempt from the Act unless they are occupied by Her Majesty in right of the Duchy of Lancaster or occupied by the possessor of the Duchy of Cornwall.

Section 20 Interpretation

In this Act, unless the context otherwise requires, the following expressions have the meanings hereby respectively assigned to them–

Section 20: 'adjoining owner' and 'adjoining occupier'

"adjoining owner" and "adjoining occupier" respectively mean any owner and any occupier of land, buildings, storeys or rooms adjoining those of the building owner and for the purposes only of section 6 within the distances specified in that section;

It is important to understand that the reference to 'any owner' indicates the possibility of there being more than one adjoining owner or occupier of land or premises adjoining that of the building owner. It could include owners and occupiers whose premises do not actually abut those of the building owner but may be directly or indirectly affected by his proposed work, for example, owners or occupiers of upper storey flats above a ground floor flat needing to be underpinned.

The reference to Section 6 makes clear that the Act also includes any owners or occupiers of premises not actually adjoining but within three metres or six metres horizontal distance of the building owner's premises.

Section 20: 'appointing officer'

"appointing officer" means the person appointed under this Act by the local authority to make such appointments as are required under section 10(8);

If the two appointed surveyors cannot agree on the selection of the third surveyor they can apply for the selection to be made by the officer appointed for that purpose by the local authority administering building control in the area where the notifiable work is to be carried out.

Section 20: 'building owner'

"building owner" means an owner of land who is desirous of exercising rights under this Act;

The term 'building owner' is specific and refers to a person or company or to an organisation desirous of executing work that is notifiable under the Act; the description must also comply with the applicable criteria defining 'owner' in Section 20.

It is essential that correct information is entered into statutory notices or awards, and it would be prudent for an adjoining owner or his appointed surveyor to confirm, usually through the Land Registry, that the building owner has good title to his premises and thus has the right to serve notice in his name and to proceed with the work.

Section 20: 'foundation'

"foundation", in relation to a wall, means the solid ground or artificially formed support resting on solid ground on which the wall rests;

Mostly foundations are of concrete, reinforced or otherwise, and usually the foundations of traditionally built brick walls will have brick offset footings to distribute the load onto the concrete base. The combination of the constituent materials does not invalidate the description; not only the concrete but the whole of the composite base is considered to be the foundation of the wall.

It is obvious that the bottom of the simple foundation referred to above and in Sections 6(1)(b) and 6(2)(b) is the bottom of the concrete base of the foundation of the adjoining owner's building. When the building owner is proposing to use piles, the lowest part of the pile itself will be the bottom of the excavations on the building owner's premises.

Section 20: 'owner' (a)–(c)

"owner" includes–

(a) a person in receipt of, or entitled to receive, the whole or part of the rents or profits of land;

(b) a person in possession of land, otherwise than as a mortgagee or as a tenant from year to year or for a lesser term or as a tenant at will;

(c) a purchaser of an interest in land under a contract for purchase or under an agreement for a lease, otherwise than under an agreement for a tenancy from year to year or for a lesser term;

An 'owner' can be a person, company or corporate body receiving or entitled to receive all or part of the rental income or profits of premises, and the title 'owner' includes the freeholder of the premises, leaseholder, subleaseholder, tenant or subtenant and any of those in possession of a tenancy of a term of more than a year. It should also be noted that someone who receives rent from subletting premises which are occupied under the terms of a 'shorthold' tenancy might also qualify as an 'owner' rather than as an occupier.

Purchasing or acquiring a lease on a property will confer the title of 'owner' once contracts have been exchanged and, if the 'owner' is the building owner, will give him entitlement to serve notice to carry out work authorised by the Act or, if an adjoining owner, will give him entitlement to receive notice of the building owner's proposals.

Responsibility for giving mandatory notice, and the consequences arising from its service, remain with the building owner, and so, should there be a change of building owner during the currency of the notice, the notice will be voided and new notice must be given to adjoining owners, and matters must be started afresh.

The Act does not require a building owner to serve any new or additional notice when a change of ownership is from one adjoining owner to a successor in title. It is usual to expect that the new adjoining owner will have been apprised by his predecessor of his status in the matter, but in any event he is bound by the notice served on the original adjoining owner.

Section 20: 'party fence wall'

> "party fence wall" means a wall (not being part of a building) which stands on lands of different owners and is used or constructed to be used for separating such adjoining lands, but does not include a wall constructed on the land of one owner the artificially formed support of which projects into the land of another owner;

A fence wall or boundary wall is party when its thickness is astride the line of junction of land of different owners; it cannot be thus defined when it is a wall to a building.

Section 20: 'party structure'

> "party structure" means a party wall and also a floor partition or other structure separating buildings or parts of buildings approached solely by separate staircases or separate entrances;

Party structures include walls and floors separating buildings or parts of premises accessed by separate staircases or entrances but could also be those accessed from lobbies off a common staircase or passageway.

In a multi-occupied building the walls surrounding hallways and staircases – the common parts – would normally be in the ownership of a freeholder and would be party walls where they physically separate the freeholders' premises from the premises accessed from the common parts. Similarly, structural floors between separate tenancies or adjoining owners are party structures, and a building owner intending to carry out work affecting the party structure is required to serve notice on both the adjoining owner and any others having a legal interest in it.

Figure 2 Definition of a party fence wall

'Party Fence Wall' as defined in Section 20 of the Act means a wall (not being part of a building) which separates the land of different owners, and which stands astride the boundary line.

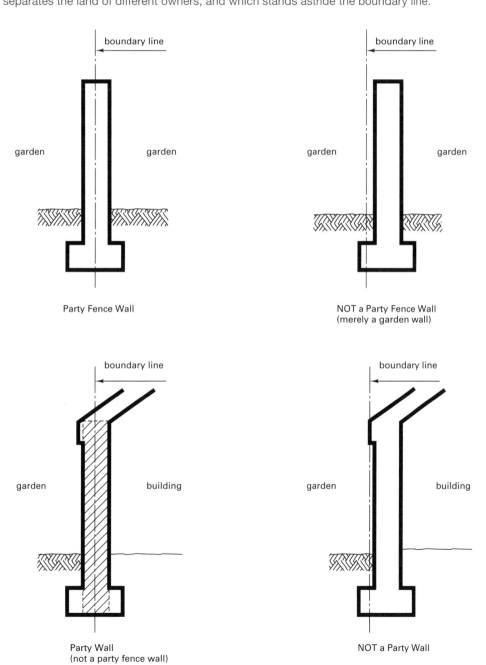

Section 20 'party wall' (a), (b)

"party wall" means–

(a) a wall which forms part of a building and stands on lands of different owners to a greater extent than the projection of any artificially formed support on which the wall rests; and

(b) so much of a wall not being a wall referred to in paragraph (a) above as separates buildings belonging to different owners;

A party wall may be defined either as in (a) a wall having its thickness, above its foundation, astride the boundary between lands of different owners, or as in (b) a wall that physically separates buildings belonging to different owners.

The boundary or line of junction separating lands of different owners may not necessarily be situated centrally within the thickness of the wall nor need its foundation be distributed equally on each owner's land but either owner can make full use of all of the wall for all its length, breadth, height and thickness in accordance with the provisions of Sections 2 and 11.

Section 20 'special foundations'

"special foundations" means foundations in which an assemblage of beams or rods is employed for the purpose of distributing any load; and

Steel reinforcement of concrete in foundations is necessary to make the two different materials act together as a single entity, and their combination makes the foundation 'special' within the terms of the Act.

Steel reinforcement used in the foundation may be of mild steel rod or joists, but using a light steel mesh that does not assist in distributing any of the load bearing on it will not make the foundation a 'special foundation'.

Section 20 'surveyor'

"surveyor" means any person not being a party to the matter appointed or selected under section 10 to determine disputes in accordance with the procedures set out in this Act.

This section refers to the appointment or selection of a surveyor as personal to him, and it specifically excludes the appointment of a party to the dispute from acting on his own behalf. The reference in Section 10(3)(c) and (5) to the possibility of the death of a surveyor or that of a surveyor becoming incapable of acting certainly disqualifies a company from being appointed.

Figure 3 Party wall – definition (a)
'Party Wall' as defined in Section 20 subsection (a) of the Act means a wall which forms part of a building, and which stands on the lands of different owners, ie astride the boundary line (though not necessarily placed centrally).

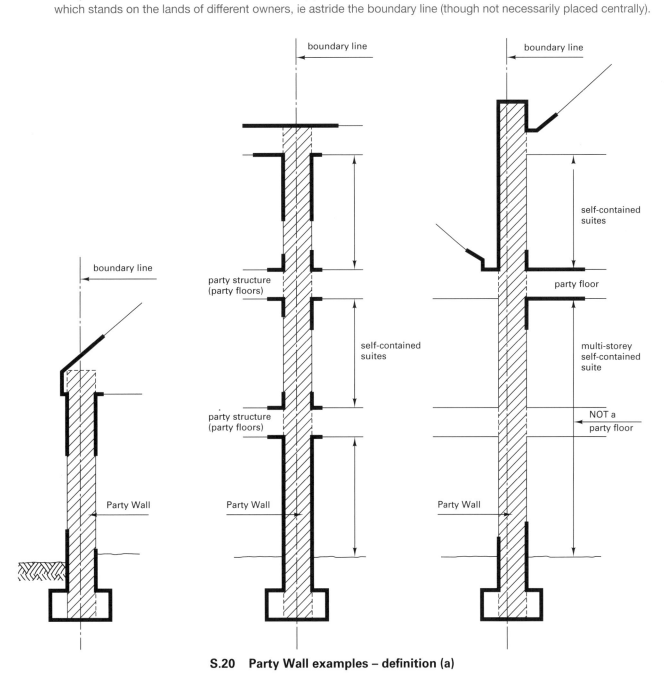

S.20   Party Wall examples – definition (a)

Figure 4 Party wall – definition (b)

'Party Wall' as defined in Section 20 subsection (b) of the Act means that portion of a wall which separates the buildings of different owners.

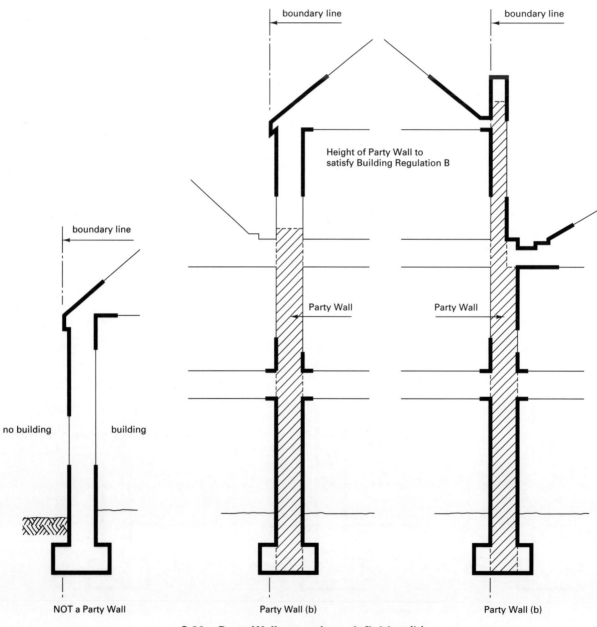

S.20   Party Wall examples – definition (b)

Although the Act does not require that the appointment must be of someone who is qualified in any particular discipline, it is obvious that a general understanding of building construction is required together with a working knowledge of the procedures of the Act.

The surveyor is appointed to resolve the dispute between the parties and he must do this in an entirely impartial manner.

While the appointed surveyor is to act impartially it has also been considered that the degree of impartiality should not be such as to disregard the interests of the party that appointed him. An architect has a similar remit in administering the traditional standard form of building contract when he is required to act in a fair and unbiased way and must hold the balance between his client who employs him and his client's contractor.

Section 21 Other statutory provisions

(1) The Secretary of State may by order amend or repeal any provision of a private or local Act passed before or in the same session as this Act, if it appears to him necessary or expedient to do so in consequence of this Act.

(2) An order under subsection (1) may–

    (a) contain such savings or transitional provisions as the Secretary of State thinks fit;

    (b) make different provision for different purposes.

(3) The power to make an order under subsection (1) shall be exercisable by statutory instrument subject to annulment in pursuance of a resolution of either House of Parliament.

General 22 Short title, commencement and extent

(1) This Act may be cited as the Party Wall etc. Act 1996.

(2) This Act shall come into force in accordance with provision made by the Secretary of State by order made by statutory instrument.

(3) An order under subsection (2) may–

    (a) contain such savings or transitional provisions as the Secretary of State thinks fit;

    (b) make different provision for different purposes.

(4) This Act extends to England and Wales only.

Preparing an Award

Preparing an Award

The prime purpose of appointing a party wall surveyor is to resolve disputes between owners. The determination of disputes is effected by an agreed and legally binding document in the form of a party wall award. This book shows what an award might include, how it should be structured, and how it relates to the requirements of the Act.

Two examples of awards are also given, the first where the parties have concurred in the appointment of an agreed surveyor, and the second where the parties have each appointed a surveyor.

When a dispute has arisen, or is deemed to have arisen, an owner may not act for himself in the matter but is obliged to appoint a surveyor to act on his behalf. It is the duty of the surveyor to act impartially and to ensure, as far as is reasonable, that a resolution of the dispute can be achieved in accordance with the provisions of the Act.

Section 20 gives several definitions of 'owner', and it is important that surveyors acting for owners named in an award have correct information in establishing and perhaps determining adjoining interests. Only an owner legally entitled to exercise his rights under the Act can appoint the surveyor. The appointment is personal to the surveyor, is made under statute, and may not be rescinded by either party to the dispute.

An architect whose practice is engaged in providing architectural services on a contract might be well placed to provide the party wall surveyor services needed for the same contract. In this situation, appointment as party wall surveyor must be separate from any other contract involving agency on behalf of the client and the appointment must comply with the provisions of Section 10 of the Act.

This would be in a personal capacity, and architects should take care to obtain a separate letter of formal appointment which includes paragraphs such as the following.

Letter from building owner to appoint an Architect as Party Wall Surveyor

---

... (address of property concerned) ...
Party Wall etc. Act 1996

I/We hereby authorise you to sign, issue and receive any notices in connection with the works proposed at the above address.

In the event of a dispute arising, we appoint you <name> as my/our party wall surveyor in accordance with Section 10 of the above Act and authorise you to make any necessary appointments on my/our behalf.

Letter from adjoining owner to appoint an architect as party wall surveyor

> ... (address of property concerned) ...
> Party Wall etc. Act 1996
>
> I/We authorise you to sign, issue and receive any notices relating to Party Wall etc. Act 1996 matters which affect my/our property. I/We appoint you <name> to act as a party wall surveyor in accordance with Section 10 of the above Act.

Who prepares the award

Where both the building owner and the adjoining owner concur in the appointment of an agreed surveyor, there is no requirements under the Act to appoint any other party wall surveyor. The agreed surveyor will settle by award the matters in dispute, and the award will be conclusive, although subject to appeal as for any award.

Where the building owner and the adjoining owner each decide to appoint their own surveyor, then the first duty of the two surveyors appointed under Section 10 of the Act is formally to select the third surveyor. The selection must be in writing, and it is usual for the building owner's surveyor to suggest the names of three surveyors for the adjoining owner's surveyor to consider. The adjoining owner's surveyor will usually agree with the building owner's surveyor on the selection of one of the three. The third surveyor will probably be known to both surveyors as someone experienced in matters concerned with party wall disputes.

If the two surveyors cannot agree on the choice of the third surveyor, or if for some reason he is unwilling or unable to act, they might agree that another third surveyor should be selected by the appointing officer of the local authority administering the building regulations for the area where the work is to be carried out. Where a party to the dispute is a local authority and the two surveyors cannot agree on the choice of the third surveyor, then an application by either surveyor may be made to the Secretary of State, who will independently make the selection of the third surveyor.

There is no need to notify the third surveyor of his selection. If he is not called upon to act in the dispute he will probably never know of it. However, it is advisable to check his general availability, and it would be in the owners' interests to ascertain what his scale of fees would be if he were to be called upon to join an appointed surveyor in making an award or, if necessary, to make his own award.

Where several adjoining owners are involved, each must respond in writing to a notice from the building owner, and either agree to the proposals or indicate dissent. If there is no reply to the notice within a period of 14 days from its receipt, dissent is deemed by default and surveyors must then be appointed. If under the provisions of Section 4 a counter notice has been issued and a dispute is deemed to have arisen, the adjoining owners are each required to appoint a surveyor to act for them under the provisions of Section 10 of the Act.

Where several adjoining owners are involved, and each is entitled to an individual award, they might agree on a sole surveyor to act for them all (although this is unlikely), and they may also agree with the building owner that his appointed surveyor acts as the agreed surveyor. The appointment of an agreed surveyor in these circumstances is unlikely for many reasons, one being that because of the relatively short period of time allowed for responses, it is often difficult for owners to agree on a course of action.

Generally, each adjoining owner will appoint his own surveyor. This will of course mean separate and individual awards involving the building owner and each respective adjoining owner, and is likely to be an expensive business. Every effort should be made to encourage adjoining owners to be pragmatic and recognise that their joint interests will usually be best served by appointing one surveyor to act for them all.

Structure of the award

The heading of the award should refer to the specific provisions of the Party Wall etc. Act 1996 under which the award is prepared by the surveyors. This will depend on the nature of the dispute and relate to the statutory notices previously served.

Recitals will rehearse the important facts underlying the dispute and confirm the identity of the surveyors appointed under Section 10, who are thereby authorised to resolve the dispute and make an award. For example:

An Award

**Under the provisions of Section 2 of the
PARTY WALL etc. ACT 1996
To be served on the appointing owners under Section 10(14)**

Whereas

....

(hereinafter referred to as the building owner)

an owner within the meaning of the said Act of the premises known as

....

did on the .... day of ....

serve upon ....
(hereinafter referred to as the adjoining owner)

an owner within the meaning of the Act, or the adjoining premises known as

....

notice of his intention to exercise the rights given to him by the
Party Wall etc. Act 1996 Section 2(2)(a)(b)(c)(d)(e)(f)(g)(h)(i)(j)(k)(l)(m)(n)*
By executing works as more particularly defined in the notice.
* *delete as appropriate*

and a dispute has arisen

And Whereas

the building owner has appointed

....

to act as his surveyor,

and the adjoining owner has appointed

....

to act as his surveyor

Where two surveyors have been appointed, it is a duty of the two surveyors to forthwith select a third surveyor. In such cases, the recitals to the award might be extended as follows.

And Whereas

The said two surveyors so appointed have selected

....

to act as third surveyor in accordance with the provisions of the said Act, and

in the event of his being unable or unwilling to act and they being unable jointly to agree upon a substitute, they have agreed that another third surveyor shall be selected by the

Appointing officer of ....

The first recital of the award formally sets out the information necessary to identify the owners and their premises and the works that the building owner intends to carry out, for example in accordance with Section 6, or in accordance with Section 2. It also states the date on which a notice was served on the adjoining owner. From this the inference is drawn that, from the date of the notice, work on site may not start before a period of one month has elapsed in the case of adjacent excavations and construction, or two months in the case of work to a party wall.

Following the recitals, the surveyors set out their award in an itemised format, typically including the following:

1. Brief reference to the salient facts, the evidence considered and those documents which constitute part of the award.

2. Proposed work which may be undertaken under the terms of the award.

3. Restrictions on any deviation from the work as described in the award.

4. Conditions which are to apply to the carrying out of the proposed work.

5. Rights of access during the carrying out of the proposed work.

6. Undertakings that work will conform to the terms of the award, CDM Regulations and be to the reasonable satisfaction of the surveyors.

7. Imposed limitations of time and working hours.

8. Surveyor's fees, and the authorisation to make further Awards where necessary.

Finally, the award agreed by the surveyors is dated, signed and witnessed. It is served on the owners forthwith in accordance with the procedures in Section 10(14), or in the case of an award made by a third surveyor Section 10(15).

Letter to accompany the signed award when delivered to the owners

> ... (address of property concerned) ...
>
> Party Wall etc. Act 1996
>
> I enclose herewith the building /adjoining owner's copy of the signed award concerned with the works to be carried out at the above address.
>
> I notify you that this is a legal document and if you disagree with its provisions you may, in accordance with Section 10(17) of the above Act, appeal to the county court within 14 days of your receipt of the award.

The award may have a limited life where this is stated in the document, and although subject to the rights of appeal under Section 10(17) of the Act, it is to be otherwise regarded as conclusive.

Detail of the award

Following a final recital, the appointed surveyors set out their decisions in the itemised format previously described.

The first two paragraphs of an award are usually of particular significance in that they put the document into context, and go on to describe in some detail the work which is authorised under the terms of the award.

Paragraph 1

Now We,

being two of the three surveyors so appointed and selected, and the said premises having been inspected, DO HEREBY AWARD AND DETERMINE as follows:

1(a) That the wall separating the building owner's and the adjoining owner's premises is deemed to be a party wall within the meaning of the Act.

(b) That the said wall as described in the attached schedule of condition is sufficient for the present purposes of the adjoining owner.

(c) That the schedule of condition dated .... attached hereto and signed by us the said two surveyors forms part of this award.

(d) That the drawings numbered .... attached hereto and signed by us, the said two surveyors, form part of this award.

(e) That the method statement concerning the Construction (Design and Management) Regulations 2007 relating to:
   (i) effecting resin injection repairs
   (ii) provision of an injected chemical damp-proof course
   (iii) underpinning sequences and safety procedures

   attached hereto and signed by us the said two surveyors forms part of this award.

Subparagraph (a)

This describes the siting of the properties and the physical and structural relationships of one to the other. There is an implied description of where the boundary might be found in relation to an independent building standing close to it, or in relation to the party wall.

Subparagraph (b)

This refers to such things as the gable end of the premises or the party wall, as being sufficient for the present purposes of the adjoining owner. This is a tacit acknowledgement that the adjoining owner has no interest or liability in contributing to any of the costs of the building owner's proposed works, and that the party wall or adjoining premises are not in a condition that might require the adjoining owner to pay for any remedial work in addition to the works proposed by the building owner.

Subparagraph (c)

Before work begins on site, the surveyors should agree a schedule of condition which accurately describes any areas of the adjoining owner's property that might be adversely affected by the proposed works.

Note that it is not mandatory to attach a schedule of condition to the award, and the Act does not require one to be taken. However, since the substance of Sections 2(3)–(7) is concerned with making good the adjoining owner's premises from damage resulting from the building owner's works, it makes sense to agree the condition of those areas most likely to be affected and to include a schedule in the award.

The schedule should be concise, with cracks and defects carefully noted, although no comment should be made as to what has caused them, unless this is self-evident. Hairline cracks should be described as such, with other crack widths measured and recorded and, if required, their orientation plotted on a drawing.

Photographs may be taken as additional records of the condition of the adjoining property, but they are not a reliable substitute for a written record and can be a costly and perhaps unnecessary addition to award documentation.

Under Section 8(1), rights of entry, the building owner is allowed to remove furniture and fittings as necessary. Before doing so, he should make a careful record of items likely to be affected by the building operations.

Subparagraph (d)

Drawings are required to accompany notices served under Section 3(1)(b) concerning special foundations, and Section 6(6) concerning adjacent excavation and construction. The drawings should clearly describe the intended work, and should augment and amplify the drawings that accompany the notice giving the information required by the Act.

The amount of detail provided about the proposed work is typically only the minimum required for compliance with the Act, and an adjoining owner's surveyor will often want a fuller description before an award can be settled. This is best done by drawings specifically produced to describe the intended works. Drawings should preferably be A4, or folded to A4 size, and put into a wallet bound to the award. It is important to make sure that the drawings do not become separated from the award document itself.

Subparagraph (e)

Since the introduction of the Construction (Design and Management) Regulations 1994, revised 2007, it has become common practice to include in the award the various method statements that could have been required by the planning supervisor for the project when the health & safety plan was being compiled. These are often lengthy and, like the drawings, should be securely attached to the award. The appointed surveyors should sign all the drawings and documents attaching to and forming part of the award.

Paragraph 2

2 That on the service of the signed award but before the expiration of the period prescribed by the said Act for service of the notice in respect of which the dispute has arisen, the building owner shall be free if he so chooses but shall be under no obligation to carry out the following works:

(a) Resin grouting and brick stitching to the fractures in the party wall.

(b) Cutting into the party wall to provide toothing and bonding for a new brick pier in the rear wall at ground floor level.

(c) Cutting into the party wall for the insertion of a concrete padstone and RSJ.

(d) Excavating adjacent to the party wall, cutting off footings and foundations, and underpinning as necessary to a minimum depth of 1.2 m or as required by the building inspector.

(e) Carrying out necessary demolition and reconstruction of defective chimney breasts and stacks together with repairs and rebuilding of defective parapets and copings, including the provision of new lead flashings and weatherings at both sides of the party wall.

(f) Drilling into the party wall at near ground floor level to provide an injected chemical damp-proof course.

The form of wording used in many awards seems to imply that only after 14 days have elapsed from receipt of an award is the building owner permitted to proceed with his works on site. The Act does not say so: this is something that the surveyors determine. However, Section 10(17) of the Act gives the right to either of the parties in dispute to appeal to the county court against the award, and the county court may rescind the award or modify it as it thinks fit.

An appeal to the county court must be made within 14 days from the day that the signed award is served on the owners. The award is conclusive, and although it would be prudent for a building owner to allow 14 days to elapse before being satisfied that the adjoining owner has not appealed the award and that work can proceed on site, two weeks of additional delay to a contract may be unacceptable. If the building owner decides to start work immediately on receipt of the signed award, he is taking a calculated risk, but in relation to the notice served, he may only start work if the relevant statutory period has run. He can only start earlier with the written agreement of the adjoining owner.

Subparagraphs (a)–(f)

These give the particulars of the extent of the works proposed by the building owner. Although the appointed surveyors are able to determine the right, time and manner of executing the works, the Act does not empower them to agree any works not specifically described in the notice(s) served on the adjoining owner.

Case Study A

Case Study A: Green Street, Tring

An award by an agreed surveyor

John Smith of Tring wishes to undertake work on his property which involves the placing of ground beams and piles. A notice has been served on the adjoining owner, New World Housing Association, as required by Section 6 of the Act, because of the proximity of the boundary to the proposed work.

The notice was sent together with a letter of explanation (see below) and New World Housing Association responded with a formal notice of dissent requesting that the foundations of the south wall of its building should be underpinned or strengthened, or otherwise safeguarded.

The notices were served using the model forms in this book. A dispute has therefore arisen, and the parties are required under Section 10 to appoint surveyors. Sensibly, the parties concurred in the appointment of an agreed surveyor, a Mr R S Jay. His award is reproduced in full, together with the accompanying drawings which form part of it. Explanatory notes on the award follow it.

All names and addresses used in this example are fictitious and are not intended to represent or bear resemblance to any living persons or places.

Letter to accompany a party structure notice or a
notice of adjacent excavation and construction

Under the provisions of the Party Wall etc. Act 1996 <name of building
owner(s)> are obliged to serve you with the attached notice of his/their*
intention to carry out work which is likely to affect your property.

This letter is to explain in less formal terms that if you disagree with any of the
proposed works, the law requires that you appoint a surveyor to safeguard your
interests, and his fee, in all normal circumstances, will be paid by the building
owner. Naturally the building owner will also be responsible for making good
any damage that the work may cause.

I would be grateful to know whether or not you agree to the proposed work, and,
if you are intending to appoint a surveyor to act for you, would ask you to let me
know who this will be. Under the provisions of Sections 5 and 10(1), (a) and (b)
of the Party Wall etc. Act 1996, should you disagree with the works proposed,
you are entitled to appoint me as the 'agreed surveyor', whereby there would
be no necessity for you to appoint any other surveyor. All surveyors appointed
under the provisions of the above Act must act impartially between the parties so
as to settle matters, and the appointment of an agreed surveyor does not prejudice
an owners' rights or entitlements.

Within 14 days of receipt of the notice, please complete and return the
accompanying acknowledgement form in the enclosed prepaid envelope. Would
you please also tell me if you know of any other person having a legal interest in
your property, e.g. landlord or tenant, who should also receive notice.

If you disagree with the building owner's proposals or fail to indicate your
consent within 14 days of receiving this notice, the Act states that a dispute has
arisen or is deemed to have arisen. Under these circumstances you may wish to
concur in the appointment of <building owner's proposed surveyor> as an agreed
surveyor who will act impartially in matters affecting you and the building
owner. If you do not wish to concur, then the Act requires you to separately
appoint a surveyor.

I would be pleased to explain the proposed work in further detail and the
formalities required by legislation.

*Delete as appropriate.

Notice	**Adjacent excavation and construction**

To *(adjoining owner)*:   Name: *New World Housing Association*

Address: *21 Station Road, Pinner, Middx.*

From *(building owner)*:   Name: *John Smith*

Address: *8 Green Street, Tring, Hertfordshire.*

Under the Party Wall etc. Act 1996 Section 6

As building owner of the land and premises known as

8 Green Street, Tring, Hertfordshire.

I/~~WE~~ HEREBY GIVE YOU NOTICE THAT

- ~~I/We intend to build within 3 metres of your building and to a level lower than the bottom of your foundations;~~
  ~~OR~~
- I/~~We~~ intend to build within 6 metres of your building and to a level as defined in Section 6(2) of the Act.

- The proposed works are described below/shown on the attached drawings etc. (ref):
  drawing nos 09/28/28, 29 and 30

  Excavating the site at 8 Green Street to reduce levels.

  Placing continuous flight auger piles and excavating for and casting ground beams to form the foundations to the structure of the proposed three-storey block of flats.

- I/~~We~~ propose/~~do not propose/~~ to ~~underpin, strengthen or otherwise~~ safeguard the foundations of your building at my/~~our~~ expense.

- It is intended to commence the work after one month, on or about

  (date)   *01/06/2009*

- In the event of matters which require to be resolved, I/~~we~~ will appoint as my/~~our~~ surveyor.

  (name)   *R S Jay RIBA*

  (address)   *The Studio, 17 Aston Gardens, London N1 3PQ.*

Signed _____   Date *01/07/2009*

* Delete as appropriate   (Owner/~~Owner's Agent~~)*
John Smith

Acknowledgement of receipt of notice	**Adjacent excavation and construction**

To (*building owner*):   Name: *John Smith*

Address: *8 Green Street, Tring, Hertfordshire.*

From (*adjoining owner*):   Name: *New World Housing Association*

Address: *21 Station Road, Pinner, Middx.*

Under the Party Wall etc. Act 1996 Section 6

As adjoining owner of the land and premises known as

10/16 Green Street, Tring, Hertfordshire.

and with reference to the Notice of Adjacent Excavation and Construction

concerning   *8 Green Street, Tring, Hertfordshire.*   dated   *01/06/2009*

I/WE HEREBY GIVE YOU NOTICE THAT

- ~~I/We dispute the necessity for you to underpin or strengthen the foundations of my/our building;~~
~~OR~~
- I/We require you to underpin or strengthen the foundations of ~~my~~/our building as described below/as shown on the attached drawings etc. (ref):

  Underpin or otherwise strengthen the foundations of the gable wall between Nos 10 and 8 Green Street.

In the event of matters which require to be resolved

- I/We concur in the appointment as agreed survey or

OR
- ~~I/we will appoint as my/our surveyor~~

  (name)   *R S Jay RIBA*

  (address)   *The Studio, 17 Aston Gardens, London N1 3PQ.*

Signed _____   Date   *10/07/2009*

* Delete as appropriate

(~~Owner~~/Owner's Agent)*
New World Housing Association

An Award

**under the provisions of Section 6 of the
Party Wall etc. Act 1996
to be served on the appointing owners under Section 10(14)**

Whereas

John Smith of 8 Green Street, Tring, Hertfordshire
(hereinafter referred to as the building owner)
an owner within the meaning of the said Act of the premises known as,
8 Green Street, Tring, Hertfordshire,

did on the first day of July 2009
serve upon New World Housing Association
of 21 Station Road, Pinner, Middlesex
(hereinafter referred to as the adjoining owner)
an owner within the meaning of the Act of the adjoining premises known as
10–16 Green Street, Tring, Hertfordshire,

notice of his intention to exercise the rights given to him by the
Party Wall etc. Act 1996 Section 6(1)(a), (b)
by executing works as more particularly defined in the notice.

And Whereas

as provided by Section 6(3) of the said Act the adjoining owner
did on the tenth day of July 2009 serve on the building owner written request that
the building owner shall at his own expense underpin or strengthen or otherwise
safeguard the foundations of the south wall of the adjoining owner's building.

and a dispute has arisen

And Whereas

the building owner and the adjoining owner have concurred in the appointment of
R S Jay RIBA, MIStructE
of The Studio, 17 Aston Gardens, London N1 3PQ.
to act as the agreed surveyor, to act impartially in these matters,
in accordance with the provisions of Section 10(1)(a) of the Act.

Now I,

the agreed surveyor so appointed having inspected the said premises, do hereby award and determine as follows:

1 (a) That 10–16 Green Street, Tring, Hertfordshire is an independent building standing close to or adjoining the boundary within the meaning of the Act.

   (b) That the said premises and particularly the gable end wall of 10–16 Green Street as described in the attached schedule of condition are sufficient for the present purposes of the adjoining owner.

   (c) That the schedule of condition dated 20 July 2009 attached hereto and signed by me the said agreed surveyor forms part of this award.

   (d) That the drawings numbered 09/28/28 and 29 and 30 attached hereto and signed by me the said agreed surveyor form part of this award.

   (e) That the method statements relating to the procedure and bay sequence of underpinning works and the provision and maintenance of access to the adjoining owner's premises during the course of the works are attached hereto and signed by me the said agreed surveyor form part of this award.

2 That on delivery of the signed award but after the expiration of the period prescribed by the said Act for service of the notice in respect of which the dispute has arisen the building owner shall be free if he so chooses but shall be under no obligation to carry out the following works:

   (a) Excavating and underpinning to a minimum depth of 2.25 m or as required by the building inspector the south gable wall of the adjoining owner's building to the reasonable satisfaction of the agreed surveyor and in accordance with the specification and details shown on drawing no. 09/28/29 attached hereto and signed by me the said Agreed Surveyor.

   (b) Demolishing the existing building at 8 Green Street and excavating to reduce ground levels.

   (c) Placing continuous flight auger piles below ground level and excavating for and casting ground beams to form the foundation to the structure of the proposed three-storey block of flats.

   The above described works will be carried out in accordance with the details shown on drawing nos 09/28/28 and 29 and 30 attached hereto and signed by me the said agreed surveyor.

3 That no material deviation from the said agreed works shall be made by the building owner without prior consultation with and prior express written agreement by the adjoining owner or by the agreed surveyor conveying such prior written agreement on behalf of the adjoining owner.

4   That if the building owner exercises the above rights he shall:

(a) Execute the whole of the aforesaid works at the sole cost of the building owner including the payment of all statutory fees.

(b) Take all reasonable precautions and provide all necessary support to uphold and retain the adjoining owner's land and buildings.

(c) Make good forthwith all structural or decorative damage to the adjoining owner's building occasioned by the said works in materials to match existing works or, if required by the adjoining owner, make payment in lieu of carrying out work to rectify the damage. The manner and timing of any making good shall be agreed between the parties or, in default of such agreement, as determined by the agreed surveyor.

(d) Hold the adjoining owner free from liability in respect of any injury to or loss of life of any person or damage to property caused by or in consequence of the execution of the said works and the cost of making any justified claims.

(e) Permit the agreed surveyor to have access to the building owner's premises at all reasonable times during the progress of the said works.

(f) Carry out the whole of the said works from the building owner's side. Where access to the adjoining owner's premises adjacent to the boundary is required, written notice of a minimum of 14 days as required by Section 8 of the said Act, shall be given.

(g) Remove any scaffolding or screens as soon as possible and clear away dust and debris from time to time as necessary and as required by the agreed surveyor.

5   That the agreed surveyor shall be permitted access to the adjoining owner's property from time to time during the progress of the works and after its completion at reasonable times after giving reasonable notice.

6   That the whole of the works referred to in this award shall be executed in accordance with the Building Regulations, the Construction (Design & Management) Regulations 2007 and any other requirements of statutory authorities, and shall be executed in a proper and workmanlike manner in sound and suitable materials in accordance with the terms of the award and to the reasonable satisfaction of the agreed surveyor.

7   That the works shall be carried through with reasonable expedition after commencement and so as to avoid any unnecessary inconvenience to the adjoining owners or occupiers and shall be restricted to between the hours of 0800 and 1730, Monday to Friday, and 0800 and 1300 Saturdays, and as regulated by the local authority. No work shall be carried out Sundays or public holidays. Works causing excessive noise or vibration shall be restricted to not more than a two-hour period each during the morning and afternoon, Monday to Friday between 0800 to 1000 and 1530 to 1730 and between 0900 to 1100 Saturdays.

8   That a copy of the signed award shall be served forthwith on each appointing owner. An unsigned copy of the award shall be retained by the agreed surveyor.

9 That the building owners shall pay the agreed surveyor's reasonable fee of £ <amount> plus VAT and disbursements in connection with the preparation of this award and for <number> subsequent inspections of the works. In the event of damage being caused or other contingencies or variations arising necessitating further inspections, a further fee shall be payable at the hourly rate of £<amount> plus VAT.

10 That I the said agreed surveyor reserve the right to make and issue any further award or awards that may be necessary, as provided in the said Act.

11 That this award shall be null and void if the permitted works are not commenced within 12 months from the date of the award.

12 That whereas I being the said agreed surveyor so appointed under the said Act refer in this award to all matters constrained by the Construction (Design & Management) Regulations 2007 and I aver and confirm that I have approved no design.

13 That nothing in this award shall be held as conferring, admitting or affecting any right to light or air or any other easement whatsoever.

14 That notwithstanding the right of appeal against the award given by Section 10(17) of the said Act this award shall be conclusive.

In Witness Whereof I have set my hand

this _____ day of _____ (month) _____ (year)

Agreed surveyor
_____

Witness
Name _____

Address _____

Occupation _____

Informative

This award gives authority to the works that are the subject of the statutory notice served on the adjoining owner on the first day of July 2009. The agreed surveyor advises the building owner that, with regard to the proposed construction works, any required endorsements to relevant insurance policies should be effected accordingly, and that the provisions and constraints of this award and all necessary information concerned with the design and execution of the said works be made known to the building owner's contractors and operatives prior to the implementation of the works on site.

Figure 5

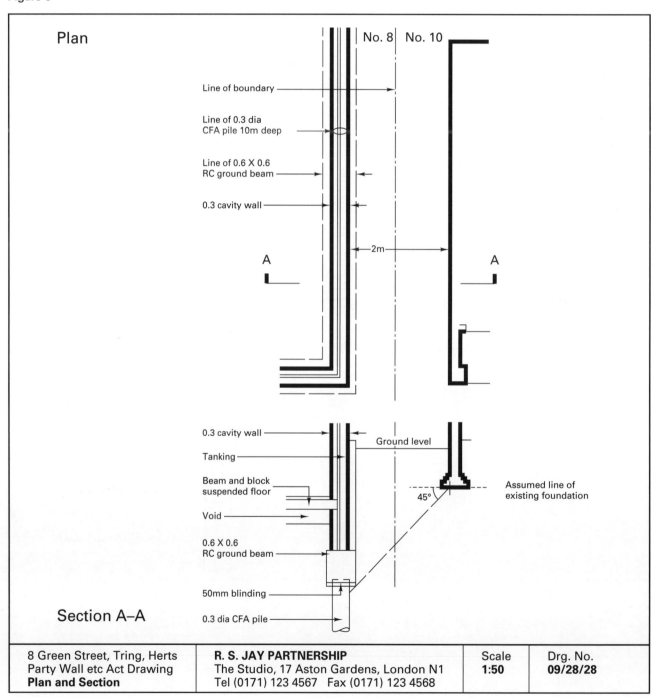

8 Green Street, Tring, Herts Party Wall etc Act Drawing **Plan and Section**	**R. S. JAY PARTNERSHIP** The Studio, 17 Aston Gardens, London N1 Tel (0171) 123 4567 Fax (0171) 123 4568	Scale **1:50**	Drg. No. **09/28/28**

Figure 6

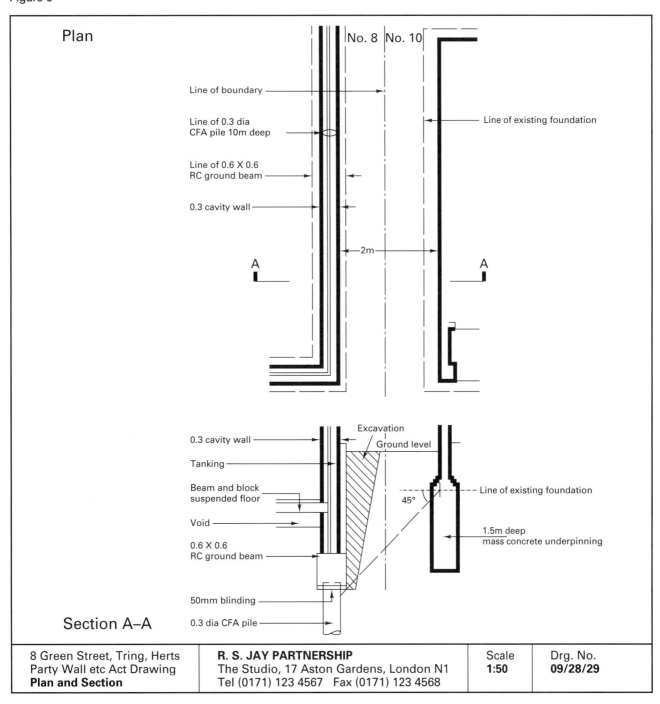

Plan

No. 8   No. 10

Line of boundary

Line of 0.3 dia
CFA pile 10m deep

Line of 0.6 X 0.6
RC ground beam

0.3 cavity wall

Line of existing foundation

←—2m—→

A   A

Section A–A

0.3 cavity wall

Tanking

Beam and block
suspended floor

Void

0.6 X 0.6
RC ground beam

50mm blinding

0.3 dia CFA pile

Excavation
Ground level

Line of existing foundation

45°

1.5m deep
mass concrete underpinning

8 Green Street, Tring, Herts Party Wall etc Act Drawing **Plan and Section**	**R. S. JAY PARTNERSHIP** The Studio, 17 Aston Gardens, London N1 Tel (0171) 123 4567 Fax (0171) 123 4568	Scale **1:50**	Drg. No. **09/28/29**

Figure 7

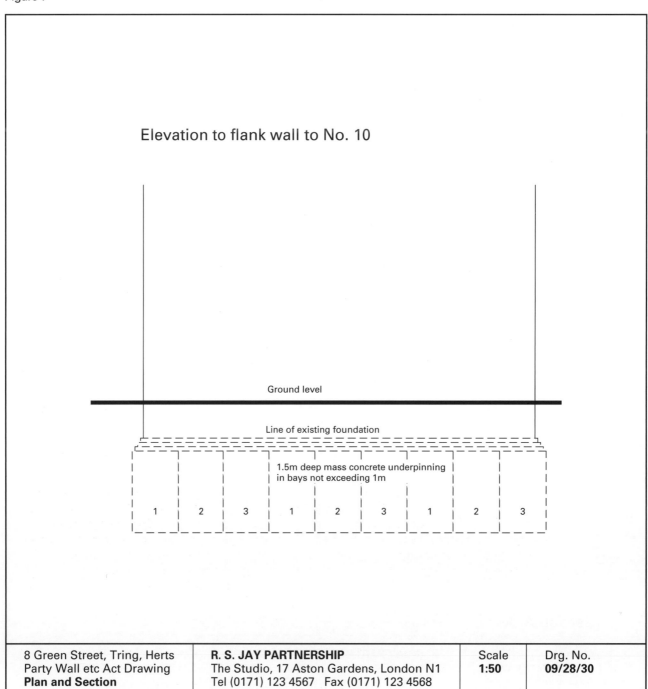

Elevation to flank wall to No. 10

Ground level

Line of existing foundation

1.5m deep mass concrete underpinning
in bays not exceeding 1m

1 2 3 1 2 3 1 2 3

8 Green Street, Tring, Herts Party Wall etc Act Drawing **Plan and Section**	**R. S. JAY PARTNERSHIP** The Studio, 17 Aston Gardens, London N1 Tel (0171) 123 4567 Fax (0171) 123 4568	Scale **1:50**	Drg. No. **09/28/30**

Notes on the award

Paragraph 1

This is an important summary of the case. It needs to be adequately full and factually correct, with a list of the documents which were taken into account and which form part of the award.

Paragraph 2

Subparagraphs (a), (b)

The work proposed to be undertaken is to demolish the existing building and excavate to reduce levels, and to place continuous flight auger piles below ground level to form the foundations for ground beams supporting the superstructure of the three-storey block of flats proposed, and as shown on drawing nos 09/28/28 and 29 (Figures 5 and 6).

The notice served on the adjoining owner would have had to have stated whether there was an intention to underpin, strengthen or safeguard the foundations of the adjoining owner's building or structure. In this instance, the notice has stated safeguarding, since the structural engineers have taken the view that adjacent foundations are not prejudiced by the use of continuous flight auger piles and are therefore safeguarded. Other methods of safeguarding could include sheet piling, strutting and propping, and excavations which avoid the intersection of the line drawn at 45° from the bottom of the adjoining owner's foundation – see Section 6(1) and (2).

The building owner proposes to use continuous flight auger piles for the new work and relies on this system to safeguard the foundations of the adjoining owner's building. Although the piles are to be placed within two metres of the adjacent foundations, the building owner's proposals would appear to be reasonable.

However, the excavations for the proposed ground beams give rise for concern, despite the fact that they are to be set lower than the level of the bottom of the foundations of the adjacent building, although not intersecting the line of the angle of repose of the soil below its foundation. Excavation is not a precise art, and owing to site conditions, excavations may be made at lower levels than originally intended. In this particular case, the adjoining owner wishes to have underpinning work carried out to avoid any risk of subsidence.

Paragraph 3

The agreed surveyor may permit minor deviations and variations to the building owner's works, but if in the course of excavation it became apparent that, for instance, subsoil conditions were not as expected, or obstructions were encountered needing piles to be adjusted and offset, then an addendum award might be needed.

Paragraph 4

Subparagraph (a)

This confirms that when the building owner undertakes work for his own benefit, it will be at his sole cost. The cost of work engendered by an adjoining owner's counter notice would be shared by the owners in accordance with the provisions of Section 11.

Subparagraph (b)

The building owner is required to take all reasonable precautions and provide all necessary support to retain the adjoining owner's land and buildings during the course of the works.

Subparagraph (c)

If the building owner's works cause structural or decorative damage to the adjoining owner's building, the building owner is required to make good the damage 'forthwith'. However, this might not be good structural practice, or it might be inconvenient for one or both owners to make good damage immediately after it has occurred. For example, differential settlement is often caused by underpinning works, and it will not be in either of the owners' best interests to repair cracking caused by subsidence before being reasonably sure that structural movement has ceased, which requires the fractures to be monitored over a lengthy period of time.

Subparagraph (d)

The building owner would be well advised to take out insurance cover to indemnify the adjoining owner against claims made against him by, for example, tenants or occupiers who might be affected by the building owner's works. The surveyor may inspect the building owner's and his contractor's relevant insurance policies covering the proposed works and advice as to the necessity to take out appropriate insurance is given in the informative on the final page of the award.

Subparagraph (e)

The Surveyor will wish to check that the work being carried out at the building owner's premises accords with what has been described in the notice and in the award. This paragraph provides for access at all reasonable times.

Subparagraph (f)

The building owner will want to make all reasonable efforts to confine his works to his side of the boundary. There are many instances where this is difficult, if not impossible, to achieve.

Subparagraph (g)

It is inevitable that the building owner's proposed works will result in noise, dust and inconvenience to the adjoining owner and occupiers of his premises. The award requires dust and debris to be kept to a minimum and that equipment, protective screens and scaffolding should be cleared away as soon as possible following the completion of work stages or as reasonably required by the surveyor. Sometimes, in response to a complaint by a neighbour, the local authority will intervene where a contractor has neglected his duties.

Paragraph 5

The agreed surveyor is allowed access to the adjoining owner's property from time to time, and when it might be prudent to check that the building owner's works were proceeding as set out in the award.

Paragraph 6

The works have to be carried out in compliance with the Building Regulations and the CDM Regulations. On his site visits the surveyor needs to satisfy himself that the works accord with the descriptions set out in the award.

Paragraph 7

The building owner is expected to carry out his works as speedily as possible so as to limit the disturbance and disruption suffered by the adjoining owner or occupiers.

Paragraph 8

'Forthwith' means that the signed awards must be served on the owners without delay. The surveyor will send signed copies of the award to the appointing owners. The copy of the award should be accompanied by a note to the owners informing them of their rights to appeal the award within 14 days of receipt.

Paragraphs 9 and 10

The agreed surveyor will rely on these provisions to obtain payment of his fees for preparing the award and where it becomes necessary to make further inspections or to produce addendum awards.

Paragraph 11

The wording should follow the notice in identifying the works which are the subject of the award, and which have to commence within 12 months from the date of the award and be properly progressed. The award and all its provisions are voided if the stated period is exceeded, although nothing in the Act prevents the owners from agreeing different dates.

Paragraph 12

Since the CDM Regulations 2007 affect nearly all building contracts, Awards may contain documents required by that legislation. These may be method statements, scaffolding and specialist drawings etc., produced for inclusion in the health & safety plan and generally described under the CDM Regulations as 'designs'. Under the Party Wall etc. Act 1996, a surveyor may determine how and when permitted works may be executed, but he is not empowered to approve a design or warrant, or endorse the efficacy of the building owner's proposals.

Paragraph 13

An award may not create easements. Although the owners may have agreed to include in an award what purports to create an easement, an award containing such an obvious transgression of Section 9 of the Act would be considered unlawful and could be rescinded by the court at any time.

Paragraph 14

The award is conclusive unless it is appealed by either owner within 14 days of its receipt. After 14 days from the day of its delivery the right of appeal is lost.

In Witness Whereof etc.

Witnesses should be of age and give their residential addresses.

Case Study B

Case Study B: Kings Walk, Elstree

An award by two appointed surveyors

Amanda Bond of Elstree requires that work be carried out on her property. This will involve the party wall, and operations which fall within Section 2 of the Act, namely Section 2(2)(a) underpinning, (b) resin grouting, insertion of an RSJ, brick stitching, rebuilding parapet walls, chimney breasts and stacks etc., (f) injecting a chemical damp-proof course, (g) underpinning, (k) repairing and constructing the brickwork junctions between the party wall and the rear wall.

As required under Section 3 of the Act, a party structure notice has been served on the adjoining owners, the Fairmile Property Co. Ltd.

The adjoining owners formally acknowledge receipt of Ms Bond's notice, sent to them by her agents. In it, they have indicated that there are aspects of the proposals that they do not agree with, although they do not appear to have served a separate counter notice. Nevertheless, the acknowledgement would not preclude the issue of a counter notice, and there is clear evidence of dissent.

The adjoining owners did not find the idea of an agreed surveyor acceptable, and nominated their own surveyor. The two surveyors were able to agree an award without calling on the selected third surveyor to act, and their award is reproduced in full together with the accompanying drawings which form part of it. Explanatory notes on the award are given.

All names and addresses used in this example are fictitious and are not intended to represent or bear resemblance to any living persons or places.

Party Structure Notice

To *(adjoining owner)*:   Name: *The Fairmile Property Co Ltd*

Address: *1 Salisbury Street, Pinner, Middx.*

From *(building owner)*:   Name: *Amanda Bond*

Address: *3 Kings Walk, Elstree, Hertfordshire.*

Under the Party Wall etc. Act 1996 Section 3

As building owner of the land and premises known as

3 Kings Walk, Elstree, Hertfordshire.

and with reference to the party structure/party wall/party fence wall separating this from adjoining land and premises.

I/WE HEREBY GIVE YOU NOTICE THAT

- ~~I/We intend to exercise the right given to me/us by Section 2 of the Act to carry out the work described below/shown on the attached drawings etc. (ref):~~
  09/18/32, 33 and 34

  For description of work, see items 1 to 6 listed overleaf.

- I/~~We~~ intend to build within 6 metres of your building and to a level as defined in Section 6(2) of the Act.

- It is intended to commence the work after two months on or about

  (date)   *1 September 2009*

- In the event of matters which require to be resolved, I/~~we~~ will appoint as my/~~our~~ surveyor.

  (name)   *R S Jay RIBA*

  (address)   *The Studio, 17 Aston Gardens, London N1 3PQ.*

Signed _____   Date *01/07/2007*

* Delete as appropriate   *(Owner/~~Owner's Agent~~)* *
Amanda Bond

reverse side

This is the list referred to on the face of this form.
To be read in conjunction with drawings 09/18/32, 33 and 34.

1   Resin grouting and brick stitching to the fractures in the party wall.

2   Cutting into the party wall to provide toothing and bonding for a new brick pier in the rear wall at ground floor level.

3   Cutting into the party wall for the insertion of a concrete padstone and RSJ.

4   Excavating adjacent to the party wall, cutting off footings and foundations and underpinning as necessary to a minimum depth of 1.2 m or as required by the building inspector.

5   Carrying out necessary demolition of chimney breasts at ground floor and reconstruction of defective chimney breasts and stack together with repairs to second stack, and rebuilding of defective parapets and copings including the provision of new lead flashings at both sides of the party wall.

6   Drilling into the party wall at near ground floor level to provide an injected chemical damp-proof course.

Acknowledgement of receipt of notice

To *(building owner)*:   Name: *Amanda Bond*

                             Address: *3 Kings Walk, Elstree, Hertfordshire.*

From *(adjoining owner)*:   Name: *The Fairmile Property Co Ltd*

                             Address: *1 Salisbury Street, Pinner, Middx.*

Under the Party Wall etc. Act 1996 Section 3

I/We acknowledge receipt of this notice

3 Kings Walk, Elstree, Hertfordshire.

served by   *Amanda Bond*   dated *01/07/2009*

I/WE HEREBY GIVE YOU NOTICE THAT

- ~~I/We consent to your proposals as described in your notice or shown on the accompanying drawings,~~
  ~~OR~~
- I/We do not consent to your proposals.

In the event of matters which require to be resolved

- ~~I/We concur in the appointment as agreed survey of~~

  _____

  ~~OR~~

- I/we will appoint as ~~my~~/our surveyor

  (name)   *S T Mates FRICS*

  (address)   *STM Associates, 8 High Road, Northside Park, Barnet.*

Signed _____ Date *10/07/2007*

* Delete as appropriate

(~~Owner~~/Owner's Agent)*
The Fairmile Property Co Ltd

An Award

**under the provisions of Section 2 of the
Party Wall etc. Act 1996
to be served on the appointing owners under Section 10(14)**

Whereas

Amanda Bond
(hereinafter referred to as the building owner)
an owner within the meaning of the said Act of the premises known as
3 Kings Walk, Elstree, Hertfordshire.

did on the first day of July 2009
serve upon The Fairmile Property Co Ltd of
1 Salisbury Street, Pinner, Middlesex
(hereinafter referred to as the adjoining owner)
an owner within the meaning of the Act, of the adjoining premises known as
5–15 Kings Walk, Elstree, Hertfordshire,

notice of her intention to exercise the rights given to her by the
Party Wall etc. Act 1996 Section 2(2)(a), (b), (f), (g) and (k)
by executing works as more particularly defined in the notice.

and a dispute has arisen

And Whereas

the building owner has appointed
R S Jay RIBA MIStructE
of The Studio, 17 Aston Gardens, London N1 3PQ
to act as its surveyor

and the adjoining owner has appointed
S T Mates
of STM Associates, 8 High Road, Northside Park, Barnet N11 8YX
to act as its surveyor

And Whereas

the two surveyors so appointed have selected
O S Newlyn ARIBA
of 88 Charterhouse Street, London EC1 6TR.
to act as third surveyor in accordance with the provisions of the Act and,
in the event of his being unable or unwilling to act and they being unable jointly to
agree upon a substitute, they have agreed that another third surveyor shall be
appointed by the appointing officer of the Hertfordshire County Council.

Now We,

Being two of the three surveyors so appointed and selected, having inspected the said premises, do hereby award and determine as follows:

1 (a) That the wall separating the building owner's and the adjoining owner's premises is deemed to be a party wall within the meaning of the Act.

    (b) That the said wall as described in the attached schedule of condition is sufficient for the present purposes of the adjoining owner.

    (c) That the schedule of condition dated 20 July 2009 attached hereto and signed by us the said two surveyors forms part of this award.

    (d) That the drawings numbered 09/18/32, 33 and 34 attached hereto and signed by us the said two surveyors form part of this award.

    (e) That the method statement concerning the Construction (Design & Management) Regulations 2007 relating to;
      (i)   effecting resin injection repairs
      (ii) provision of an injected chemical damp-proof course
      (iii) underpinning sequences and safety procedures

    attached hereto and signed by us the said two surveyors forms part of this award.

2   That on the service of the signed award but not before the expiration of the period prescribed by the said Act for service of the notice in respect of which the dispute has arisen the building owner shall be free if she so chooses but shall be under no obligation to carry out the following works:

    (a) Resin grouting and brick stitching to the fractures in the party wall.

    (b) Cutting into the party wall to provide toothing and bonding for a new brick pier in the rear wall at ground floor level.

    (c) Cutting into the party wall for the insertion of a concrete padstone and RSJ.

    (d) Excavating adjacent to the party wall, cutting off footings and foundations and underpinning as necessary to a minimum depth of 1.2 m or as required by the building inspector.

    (e) Carrying out necessary demolition and reconstruction of defective chimney breasts and stacks together with repairs and rebuilding of defective parapets and copings, including the provision of new lead flashings and weatherings at both sides of the party wall.

    (f) Drilling into the party wall at near ground floor level to provide an injected chemical damp-proof course.

3   That no material deviation from the said agreed works shall be made by the building owner without prior consultation with and prior express written agreement by the adjoining owner or by the adjoining owner's surveyor conveying such prior written agreement on behalf of the adjoining owner.

4   That if the building owner exercises the above rights she shall:

   (a) Execute the whole of the aforesaid works at the sole cost of the building owner including the payment of all statutory fees.

   (b) Take all reasonable precautions and provide all necessary support to uphold and retain the adjoining owner's land and buildings.

   (c) Make good forthwith all structural or decorative damage to the adjoining owner's building occasioned by the said works in materials to match existing works or, if required by the adjoining owner, make payment in lieu of carrying out work to rectify the damage. The manner and timing of any making good shall be agreed between the parties or in default of such agreement as determined by the said two surveyors.

   (d) Hold the adjoining owner free from liability in respect of any injury to or loss of life of any person or damage to property caused by or in consequence of the execution of the said works and the cost of making any justified claims.

   (e) Permit the adjoining owner's surveyor to have access to the building owner's premises at reasonable times after giving reasonable notice.

   (f) Carry out the whole of the said works from the building owner's side. Where access to the adjoining owner's premises adjacent to the boundary is required, written notice of a minimum of 14 days as required by Section 8 of the said Act, shall be given.

   (g) Remove any scaffolding or screens as soon as possible and clear away dust and debris from time to time as necessary and as required by the adjoining owner's surveyor.

5   That the building owner's surveyor shall be permitted access to the adjoining owner's property from time to time during the progress of the works and after its completion at reasonable times after giving reasonable notice.

6   That the whole of the works referred to in this award shall be executed in accordance with the Building Regulations, the Construction (Design & Management) Regulations 2007 and any other requirements of statutory authorities and shall be executed in a proper and workmanlike manner in sound and suitable materials in accordance with the terms of the award and to the reasonable satisfaction of the said two surveyors.

7 That the works shall be carried through with reasonable expedition after commencement and so as to avoid any unnecessary inconvenience to the adjoining owner or occupiers and shall be restricted to between the hours of 0800 and 1730, Monday to Friday, and 0800 and 1300 Saturdays, and as regulated by the local authority. No work shall be carried out Sundays or public holidays. Works causing excessive noise or vibration shall be restricted to not more than a two-hour period each during the morning and afternoon, Monday to Friday between 0800 and 1000 and 1530 and 1730 and between 0900 and 1100 Saturdays.

8 That a copy of the signed award shall be served forthwith on each appointing owner. An unsigned copy of the award shall be retained by the adjoining owners surveyor.

9 That the building owner shall pay the adjoining owner's surveyor's reasonable fee of £<amount> plus VAT and disbursements in connection with the preparation of this award and for <number> subsequent inspections of the works. In the event of damage being caused or other contingencies or variations arising necessitating further inspections a further fee shall be payable at the hourly rate of £<amount> plus VAT.

10 That we the said two surveyors reserve the right to make and issue any further award or awards that may be necessary, as provided in the said Act.

11 That this award shall be null and void if the permitted works are not commenced within 12 months from the date of the award.

12 That whereas we being the said two surveyors so appointed under the said Act refer in this award to all matters constrained by the Construction (Design & Management) Regulations 2007 and we aver and confirm that we have approved no design.

13 That nothing in this Award shall be held as conferring, admitting or affecting any right to light or air or any other easement whatsoever.

14 That notwithstanding the right of appeal against the award given by Section 10(17) of the said Act this award shall be conclusive.

In Witness Whereof we have set our hands

this _____ day of _____ (month) _____ (year)

**Surveyor to the
building owner**
_____

Witness
Name _____

Address _____

Occupation _____

**Surveyor to the
adjoining owner**
_____

Witness
Name _____

Address _____

Occupation _____

Informative

This award gives authority to the works that are the subject of the statutory
notice served on the adjoining owner on the first day of July 2009. The said two
surveyors advise the building owner that with regard to the proposed construction
works any required endorsements to relevant insurance policies should be
effected accordingly and that the provisions and constraints of this award and all
necessary information concerned with the design and execution of the said works
be made known to the building owner's contractors and operatives prior to the
implementation of the works on site.

Figure 8

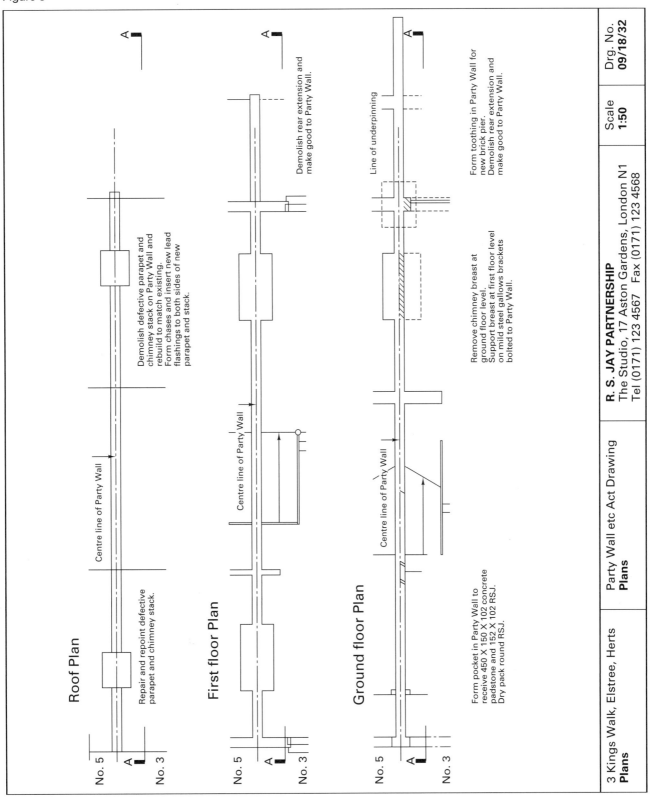

Roof Plan

Centre line of Party Wall

Demolish defective parapet and chimney stack on Party Wall and rebuild to match existing. Form chases and insert new lead flashings to both sides of new parapet and stack.

Repair and repoint defective parapet and chimney stack.

No. 5

A

No. 3

First floor Plan

Centre line of Party Wall

Demolish rear extension and make good to Party Wall.

No. 5

A

No. 3

Ground floor Plan

Centre line of Party Wall

Line of underpinning

Form toothing in Party Wall for new brick pier. Demolish rear extension and make good to Party Wall.

Remove chimney breast at ground floor level. Support breast at first floor level on mild steel gallows brackets bolted to Party Wall.

Form pocket in Party Wall to receive 450 X 150 X 102 concrete padstone and 152 X 102 RSJ. Dry pack round RSJ.

No. 5

A

No. 3

| 3 Kings Walk, Elstree, Herts **Plans** | Party Wall etc Act Drawing **Plans** | **R. S. JAY PARTNERSHIP** The Studio, 17 Aston Gardens, London N1 Tel (0171) 123 4567   Fax (0171) 123 4568 | Scale **1:50** | Drg. No. **09/18/32** |

Figure 9

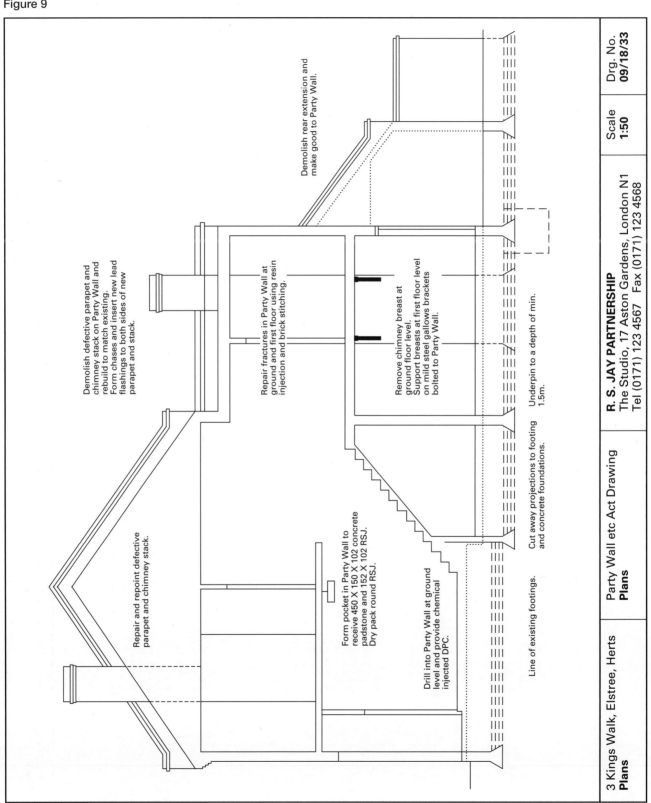

Demolish rear extension and make good to Party Wall.

Demolish defective parapet and chimney stack on Party Wall and rebuild to match existing. Form chases and insert new lead flashings to both sides of new parapet and stack.

Repair fractures in Party Wall at ground and first floor using resin injection and brick stitching.

Remove chimney breast at ground floor level. Support breasts at first floor level on mild steel gallows brackets bolted to Party Wall.

Repair and repoint defective parapet and chimney stack.

Underpin to a depth of min. 1.5m.

Cut away projections to footing and concrete foundations.

Form pocket in Party Wall to receive 450 X 150 X 102 concrete padstone and 152 X 102 RSJ. Dry pack round RSJ.

Line of existing footings.

Drill into Party Wall at ground level and provide chemical injected DPC.

| 3 Kings Walk, Elstree, Herts
Plans | Party Wall etc Act Drawing
Plans | **R. S. JAY PARTNERSHIP**
The Studio, 17 Aston Gardens, London N1
Tel (0171) 123 4567   Fax (0171) 123 4568 | Scale
1:50 | Drg. No.
09/18/33 |

Figure 10

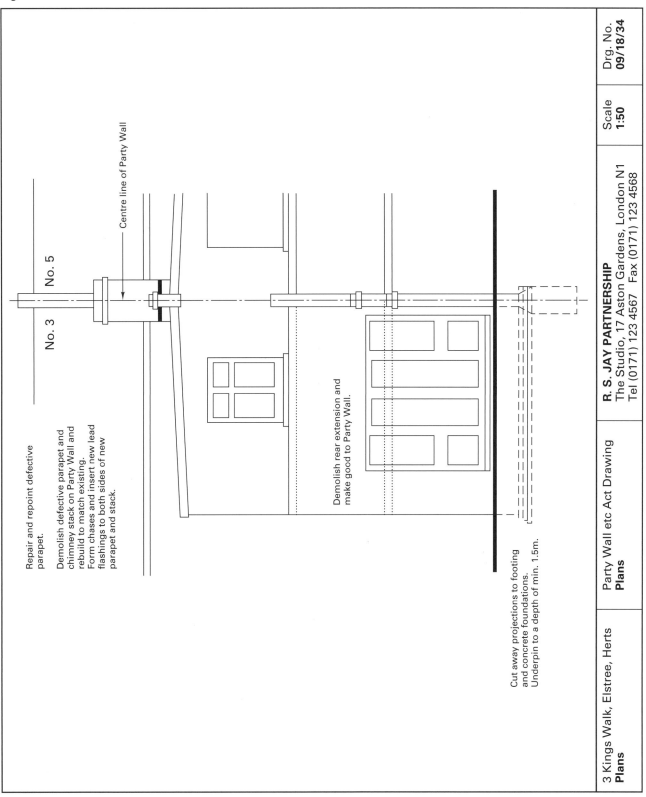

Centre line of Party Wall

No. 5

No. 3

Repair and repoint defective parapet.

Demolish defective parapet and chimney stack on Party Wall and rebuild to match existing.
Form chases and insert new lead flashings to both sides of new parapet and stack.

Demolish rear extension and make good to Party Wall.

Cut away projections to footing and concrete foundations.
Underpin to a depth of min. 1.5m.

| 3 Kings Walk, Elstree, Herts **Plans** | Party Wall etc Act Drawing **Plans** | **R. S. JAY PARTNERSHIP** The Studio, 17 Aston Gardens, London N1 Tel (0171) 123 4567 Fax (0171) 123 4568 | Scale **1:50** | Drg. No. **09/18/34** |

Notes on the Award

Paragraph 1

This is an important summary of the case. It needs to be adequately full and factually correct, with a list of the documents which were taken into account and which form part of the award.

Paragraph 2

Paragraph 2 itemises the building owner's proposed works. Where this involves the party wall, drawings should always be produced to describe the work in detail. These may be used by the contractor carrying out the work.

Paragraph 3

The adjoining owner's surveyor may permit minor deviations and variations to the building owner's works, but if in the course of excavation it became apparent that, for instance, subsoil conditions are not as expected, or obstructions were encountered needing piles to be adjusted and offset, then the agreement of the adjoining owner's surveyor will have to be obtained.

The surveyors should keep notes of all variations, however minor. If they increase substantially, an addendum award might be needed to cover the extra work and the continuing involvement of the appointed surveyors.

If variations or deviations include material changes from the proposals contained in the notice then, unless he has written authority from his appointing owner, the adjoining owner's surveyor may not agree them; new notices have to be issued. Major delay can be avoided if the adjoining owner agrees to waive notice and allows the surveyors to continue to operate on the basis of their original appointments.

Paragraph 4

Subparagraph (a)

This confirms that when the building owner undertakes work for her own benefit it will be at her sole cost. The cost of work engendered by an adjoining owner's counter notice would be shared by the owners in accordance with the provisions of Section 11.

Subparagraph (b)

The building owner is required to take all reasonable precautions and provide all necessary support to retain the adjoining owner's land and buildings during the course of the works. The adjoining owner's surveyor will need to be satisfied that any engineering proposals covering this aspect of the works are properly checked for suitability in the particular circumstances.

If the adjoining owner's surveyor is a structural or civil engineer he may be able to decide for himself that a suggested method of propping or shoring will be acceptable. However, it is more usual for the adjoining owner's surveyor to seek the advice of a structural engineer before agreeing the building owner's proposals. Whatever is awarded and determined by the surveyors it will not relieve the building owner of personal liability for damage resulting from the works.

Subparagraph (c)

If the building owner's works cause structural or decorative damage to the adjoining owner's building, the building owner is required to make good the damage 'forthwith'. However, this might not be good structural practice, or it might be inconvenient for one or both owners to make good damage immediately after it has occurred. For example, differential settlement is often caused by underpinning works, and it will not be in either owner's best interests to repair cracking caused by subsidence before being reasonably sure that structural movement has ceased, and this requires the fractures to be monitored over a lengthy period of time. In those circumstances, the two surveyors will generally determine how the matter should be dealt with and probably make and issue an addendum award to allow for repair works to be carried out at a future date. If postponing repairs is inconvenient for the adjoining owner or if he does not wish the contractors who caused the damage to carry out the repairs and prefers a cash settlement instead, the appointed surveyors will assess and agree the amount to be paid.

Subparagraph (d)

The building owner would be well advised to take out insurance cover to indemnify the adjoining owner against claims made against the Fairmile Property Co Ltd by, for example, tenants or occupiers who might be affected by the building owner's works. The adjoining owner's surveyor is entitled to ask to inspect copies of the building owner's and the contractor's insurance policies.

Subparagraph (e)

The adjoining owner's surveyor will wish to check that the work being carried out at the building owner's premises accords with what has been described in the notice and in the award. This paragraph provides for access at all reasonable times, although when the adjoining owner's surveyor wishes to inspect the adjoining premises he is not obliged to be given notice of his intentions.

Subparagraph (f)

The building owner will want to make all reasonable efforts to confine her works to her side of the boundary or party wall. There are many instances where this is difficult, if not impossible, to achieve – for example, where a building owner wishes to raise a party wall in brickwork which will form an enclosing wall to an additional storey he proposes to build on a house. The roof of the adjoining property will remain a storey below the building owner's new accommodation, which then will incorporate a new external wall to be built rising above the roof level of the adjoining property. This needs to be built and pointed using staging and scaffolding erected on the adjoining owner's side. The intention to use the adjoining owner's roof should have been stated in the notice and allowed for in the award. The building owner's programme of works should state when scaffolding is to be erected and dismantled, and include any measures necessary for compliance with the CDM regulations.

Subparagraph (g)

It is inevitable that the building owner's proposed works will result in noise, dust and inconvenience to the adjoining owner and occupiers of his premises. The award requires dust and debris to be kept to a minimum, and that equipment, protective screens and scaffolding should be cleared away as soon as possible following the completion of work stages or as reasonably required by the adjoining owner's surveyor. Sometimes, in response to a complaint by a neighbour, the local authority will intervene where a contractor has neglected his duties.

Paragraph 5

The building owner's surveyor is allowed access to the adjoining owner's property from time to time, when it might be prudent to check that the building owner's works were proceeding as set out both in the award and the notices and were not affecting the adjoining owner's premises more than could have been expected. Additions or changes in defects from those noted in the schedule of condition should be carefully recorded and agreed by the surveyors.

Paragraph 6

The works have to be carried out in compliance with the building regulations and the CDM regulations. On his site visits the adjoining owner's surveyor needs to satisfy himself that the works accord with the descriptions set out in the award, but apart from making sure that they conform with the Act and the notice, he has no duty to check their compliance with other legislation; that remains the responsibility of the building owner and her advisors.

Paragraph 7

The building owner is expected to carry out the works as speedily as possible so as to limit the disturbance and disruption suffered by the adjoining owner or occupiers. This will particularly be the case with substantial contracts, where the adjoining owner's surveyor will certainly request full details of the proposed work programme and where it may be central to the settling of the dispute that realistic commencement and completion dates are agreed and entered as express conditions of the award.

Paragraph 8

'Forthwith' means that the signed awards must be served on the owners without delay. The building owner's surveyor will usually send two signed copies of the award to the adjoining owner's surveyor, who will countersign and date both copies and return one to the building owner's surveyor. The surveyors should serve the award on their respective appointing owners on the day that the award has both signatures on each copy of the document. Each copy of the award should be accompanied by a note informing the owner of the right to appeal the award within 14 days of receipt. Although the county court may rescind or modify the award as it thinks fit, it is unlikely to question what has been described by the judge in the action of the Chartered Society of Physiotherapy v Simmonds Church Smiles, 24 January 1995 as 'an expert determination'. It would rescind an award if, for example, a surveyor had not been properly appointed or if the proposed works were not as described in the notice. An award would be rescinded if one of the parties to the dispute did not qualify as an owner as defined in Section 20.

Paragraph 9 and 10

The adjoining owner's surveyor will rely on these provisions to obtain payment of his fees for preparing the award and where it becomes necessary to make further inspections or to produce addendum awards.

Section 10(13) of the Act says that the reasonable costs incurred in making or obtaining an award or for making inspections of work to which the award relates, or any other matter arising out of the dispute, are to be paid by whichever party the surveyor or surveyors making the award determine.

The adjoining owner's surveyor has no contract with the building owner, who in normal circumstances will be responsible for all reasonable costs and fees. Therefore it is the surveyors who will determine the liability for fees, and they will award to that effect. Where a building owner withholds a payment awarded to an adjoining owner's surveyor, then providing the award has been properly signed and served on the owners, and the time allowed for appeal has elapsed, an application could be made to the magistrates' court for judgement against the building owner for recovery of a civil debt, and if the court so decides, the judgement may be entered in the award.

Paragraph 11

The wording should follow the notice in identifying the works which are the subject of the award, and which have to commence within 12 months from the date of the service of the original notice, or that date modified by the award, and be properly progressed. The award and all its provisions are voided if the stated period is exceeded, although nothing in the Act prevents the owners from agreeing different dates.

Paragraph 12

Since the CDM Regulations 2007 affect nearly all building contracts, awards may contain documents required by that legislation. These may be method statements, scaffolding and specialist drawings etc., produced for inclusion in the health & safety plan and generally described under the CDM Regulations as 'designs'. Under the Party Wall etc. Act 1996, appointed surveyors may determine how and when permitted works may be executed, but they are not empowered to approve a design or warrant, or endorse the efficacy of the building owner's proposals. The inclusion into an award of CDM documentation and the decision of the surveyors that it should be included might suggest that the surveyors themselves have approved the contents of the documentation. The statement made in paragraph 12 should make it clear that they have not.

Paragraph 13

An award may not create easements. It is unlikely, but possible, for a building owner to agree with an adjoining owner that, for example, a half round gutter may be fixed to the party wall but be positioned on the adjoining owner's side on the boundary. Any future adjoining owner would be fully entitled to exercise his rights under Section 2(2)(g) of the Act and remove the gutter if it interfered with his own proposals to build on or against the boundary. Although the owners may have agreed to include in an award what purports to create an easement, an award which contained such an obvious transgression of Section 9 of the Act would be considered unlawful and could be rescinded by the court at any time.

Paragraph 14

The award is conclusive unless it is appealed by either owner within 14 days of its receipt. After 14 days from the day of its delivery, the right of appeal is lost.

In Witness Whereof etc.

Witnesses should be of age and give their residential addresses.

Calling in the
third surveyor

Calling in the third surveyor

Immediately following their appointment, the first two surveyors must select the third surveyor, who will usually be someone senior and experienced. He is appointed to settle by award matters of difference between the parties when the first two surveyors are unable to reach agreement.

The parties to the dispute are liable for the costs arising from the third surveyor's involvement, and ideally each should be consulted by his own surveyor before the third surveyor is called in. The Act provides that either the owners or their surveyors may call on the third surveyor to determine disputed matters, but sometimes an owner prefers to try to settle matters with his neighbour before bringing in the third surveyor if this makes financial sense and might avoid delay. When an owner informs his surveyor that he wishes a third surveyor to be involved, he is exercising one of his few rights under the Act to influence or give instructions to his appointed surveyor.

The third surveyor's remit is to resolve matters in dispute between the parties, not between the surveyors. He may join one of the two surveyors in making an award, or he might disagree with both and make his own award, but he is not there to find compromise solutions.

If it is necessary for a third surveyor to be called in, the first two surveyors should restrict his work to those issues on which they disagree. He is not invited to produce an additional or alternative award, and without visiting the site and checking the schedule of condition taken and agreed by the first two surveyors, would be unable to sign their award.

The third surveyor will require copies of the documentation relating to the issues on which he is being asked to award. This might include copies of the original notices served by the owners, the signed documents relating to his own selection, copies of the letters appointing the first two surveyors, and perhaps verification of the bona fides of the owners. He will wish to be supplied with statements of the disagreement as well as the draft award, and he will probably have to go on site if the matters to be resolved are connected with construction.

Whatever has been determined in an award made by the first two surveyors, once it is agreed, it must be served forthwith on the owners.

An award made by the third surveyor alone does not have to be served on the owners until either or both pay the costs of making the award. These may include the third surveyor's fees and expenses and could include fees for a structural engineer. However, costs or payments contained in the body of the award which have been directed and determined in the resolution of the dispute between the parties would not be included.

As soon as he receives his costs for making the award, the third surveyor must serve it on the owners or on their surveyors, if they are authorised to accept service on their owners' behalf. The award is binding on the first two surveyors, but as for all awards, the third surveyor's award is subject to appeal under Section 10(17) by the owners.

If the first two surveyors accept service, the 14 days allowed for appeal against the award begins on the day they have the signed document in their hands; therefore they must immediately serve the award on their respective appointing owners to ensure that the maximum time allowed for appeal is available.

Fees

Fees

It is usual for party wall surveyors' fees to be paid by the building owner unless the adjoining owner has required or has caused additional work to be carried out subsequent, say, to serving a counter notice.

On the resolution of the matters leading to the service of an Award the building owner's surveyor will usually invoice the building owner directly and will rely for payment on any agreement he has with him as to the fees incurred in carrying out the functions of his statutory appointment or perhaps for other peripheral payments due for advising the building owner on procedural matters, especially those involving the third surveyor.

The adjoining owner's surveyor is in an entirely different position because technically he is not in contract with the building owner but with the adjoining owner and, as a consequence, his fee will be entered as a condition of the award under the provisions of Section 10(13).

In practice, surveyors rarely find it necessary to make the adjoining owner aware that when he formally dissents from a building owner's notice, and is obliged to appoint a surveyor to act on his behalf, he is also immediately responsible for any costs or expenses involved in that surveyor's appointment and, until such time as he is indemnified by the terms of the award, he is legally liable for their payment.

Due to the complex nature of the procedures leading to an award it is often difficult for a surveyor to assess with any certainty the amount of the fee that might be incurred in the matters he has been appointed to resolve and it is therefore accepted practice that fees are assessed on a time-spent basis, usually at an hourly rate; an experienced surveyor, and especially one who may be required to fee bid for his appointment, should be competent to provide a reasonable estimate of the time that he considers necessary for him to fulfil his statutory function.

It is customary for the adjoining owner's surveyor to provide information needed to substantiate the claim that his fee be awarded as submitted; the building owner's surveyor will be interested to examine the adjoining owner's surveyor's time sheets with a view to identifying items that might be questionable or those that could provoke differences of opinion between the surveyors or could give rise to an appeal against the award by either of the parties in dispute.

If the building owner's surveyor does not agree that the adjoining owner's surveyor's fee may be awarded as submitted, the matter must be referred to the third surveyor for his determination.

At the earliest opportunity the parties should be advised of an intention to involve the third surveyor and be made aware of the possibility that he may not agree with the building owner's surveyor but might award in favour of the adjoining owner's surveyor; in that event the outcome might be the building owner becoming liable for the adjoining owner's surveyor's fee as originally submitted, together with an additional fee incurred by the third surveyor for making his award.

The situation might occur also when the two surveyors had agreed the adjoining owner's surveyor's fee as submitted but the amount awarded is objected to by the building owner and, as previously stated, the award becomes subject to appeal to the county court.

There are certain issues that might arise which question the legitimacy or otherwise of the adjoining owner's surveyor's claims for fees and expenses, and these are generally concerned with the extent to which the adjoining owner's surveyor corresponds or communicates with the adjoining owner during the course of the procedures leading to the award.

The interpretation 'surveyor' (Section 20) specifically prohibits the resolution of disputed matters to be undertaken by either of the parties to the dispute but does allow them to directly call upon the third surveyor to determine issues if such requests are deemed necessary and appropriate.

The inference here is that owners are entitled to be informed of the surveyors' deliberations but not to an extent that might be considered as constituting interference, or one that would put pressure on an appointed surveyor with regard to his opinions on how the dispute should be resolved.

A surveyor may, on a general basis, keep the owner who appointed him advised of discussions and negotiations concerning the disputed matters and this may involve correspondence, telephone calls and emails etc. between them, all of which could be justification for claims for fees. In the case of the building owner's surveyor, these fees would normally be payable by the building owner on receipt of the surveyor's account; in the case of the adjoining owner's surveyor, these fees, often suggested by him to be awarded as fees payable by the building owner, are usually the responsibility of the adjoining owner and, in this regard, the building owner's surveyor should resist any misdirected claims made by the adjoining owner's surveyor and award accordingly.

There is often occasion to question the fee charged by a consultant, usually a structural engineer, who has been asked by an adjoining owner's surveyor to provide necessary expert opinion or specialist advice on the building owner's proposals. It is important to note that the consultant holds no appointment to act in the resolution of the disputed matters but is directly employed by the adjoining owner's surveyor to provide him with a service. The adjoining owner's surveyor is responsible for his consultant's fees and normally will expect to be reimbursed his expenses and disbursements.

Although it is uncommon, there also remains the possibility that a building owner might resist paying, or refuse to pay, his own appointed surveyor's fee, and in this situation the building owner's surveyor has the option either of taking legal action through the courts to recover the money or, if appropriate and not withstanding the building owner's right of appeal (Section 17), with the adjoining owner's surveyor or the third surveyor or by proceeding ex parte, making and serving an award which specifically directs his fee to be paid by the building owner.

Where an award made in the circumstances suggested above is not challenged by an appeal to the county court, and the fee remains unpaid, the Act provides for the matter to be taken to the magistrates' court where the awarded fee shall be recoverable summarily as a civil debt.

Appendix:
Access to adjoining land

Appendix: Access to adjoining land

Right of access to the land or buildings of an adjoining owner in connection with work on party walls or structures is well covered by the Party Wall etc. Act 1996. Usually the procedures laid down can be followed, and any disputes settled, without the need to bring in lawyers or involve the courts.

Access to adjoining land for other purposes is not covered by the Party Wall Act, but architects should be conversant with the provisions of the Access to Neighbouring Land Act 1992. This piece of legislation is, in the words of the full title, intended 'to enable persons who desire to carry out works to any land which are reasonably necessary for the preservation of that land to obtain access to neighbouring land to do so ...'

Someone who might otherwise be denied access by their neighbours can make application to the court for an 'access order'. This will generally mean bringing in lawyers to establish adjoining interests, to advise on the merits of an application, and to apply for a court order. Early negotiation should be tried to persuade the neighbour to agree whatever access will be necessary, but it might be easier to convince an unwilling neighbour if he is made aware of the merits of the application and that it is likely to be granted.

An access order will be made only where the court is satisfied that the works to be undertaken are reasonably necessary, cannot practicably be carried out other than from the neighbouring land, and that an unreasonable amount of interference or hardship would not be caused to the adjoining owner.

Reference to 'basic preservation to the dominant land' can include the carrying out of an inspection, the maintenance, repair, improvement, renewal or demolition of any part of a building or structure, or even work to drains etc. Although the Act is primarily concerned with works to existing property, architects may find it difficult to discern from the wording of Section 8 exactly where 'works of preservation' end and new works begin. Even building operations which are ostensibly concerned with party walls will often include both preservation and new work.

Access orders will usually specify what works are to be covered, and may impose terms and conditions such as the date or period for access, measures to be taken to protect the neighbour from damage, and inconvenience or loss of privacy etc. while work is being carried out. Access orders may be registered under the Land Charges Act 1972, and can then be binding on successors in title to the servient land. The court has the power to discharge or vary the order, or any of the terms, and also has wide powers to deal with persons who contravene or fail to comply with any requirement or condition.

The Access to Neighbouring Land Act 1992 is a relatively straightforward piece of legislation with only nine sections. Architects who undertake work where the need for such access could be critical should make themselves familiar with its provisions so as to be able to advise their clients properly. It should be noted however that this Act will not provide a remedy in every situation. For example:

- it does not cover works to party walls;

- it does not cover the use of a tower crane with an oversailing jib;

- it does not cover the provision of access to consecrated land where the law of the consistory courts of the Church of England will apply;

- it does not indicate that the owner of the servient land would not be liable for costs if opposition to an access order proved unsuccessful.

And, as already remarked, it does not unequivocally define 'works of preservation'. Section 1(4) of the Act says that 'basic preservation works' can mean 'the maintenance, repair or renewal of any part of a building or other structure comprised in, or situate on, the dominant land'. It would seem that the word 'renewal' could include the demolition and redevelopment of the major part of the structure.

The need for access to adjoining land will often occur with building operations, and architects who are extending the range of professional services they are able to offer clients will find that they sometimes have to undertake work which has traditionally been the preserve of lawyers and surveyors. For example, where scaffolding has to be placed on adjoining land, or where the jib of a tower crane is likely to oversail adjoining land, it might be necessary to secure agreement to avoid an injunction for trespass. In such cases architects might play a very useful role in negotiating licences which constitute legal agreements.

Two examples of draft licences which constitute agreement to waive rights to air space temporarily during development are included below. The first is in respect of the erection and use of scaffolding, and the second is in respect of an oversailing crane jib. As with all contracts, two copies of a licence should be engrossed and signed. One signed copy should be delivered to each of the parties to the agreement.

This Licence has been prepared by

_____

(Insert name and address of Architect's practice)

Licence   **Waive certain rights**

An Agreement by way of Licence

to waive certain rights to

_____

(Insert here ground on which scaffold will be placed, e.g. hard standing, tarmac etc.)

and air space during the development of

_____

(Insert here address of site)

development site

Whereas

in this Licence the following expressions are to have the meanings described therein:

"The Licensor"   shall mean

_____

(Insert here name of Licensor)

"The Licensor's   shall mean
Property"

_____

(Insert here address of Licensor's property)

"The Licensee"   shall mean

_____

(Insert here name of building owner/developer or contractor, as appropriate)

"The Licensee's   shall mean the land comprising the site known as
Property"

_____

(Insert here address of Licensor's site

development site shown for the purposes of identification only edged green on the plan annexed hereto ("the Plan")

"The Licensee's   shall mean the scaffolding and equipment used by the Licensee to be placed on the
Equipment"

_____

(Insert here description of ground on which scaffold is to be placed)

and extending into the air space above the Licensor's property to the extent detailed on the plan annexed hereto ("the Plan")

And Whereas

the Licensee intends to carry out work to the Licensee's property but will require the use of scaffolding and equipment (hereinafter called the Licensee's scaffolding) to facilitate the prompt completion of the said works

And Whereas

the Licensor hereby confirms that the land and the right to the air above the Licensor's property is vested in their title to the said property

Now the Licensor and the Licensee
do hereby agree
to enter into this licence as follows

1 Granting of Licence

1.1 That in consideration of the undertakings and conditions hereinafter reserved and contained, the Licensor hereby grants to the Licensee by way of Licence permission to transport, erect, install, repair, maintain, operate and dismantle with all necessary and usual ancillary works the Licensee's scaffold on the Licensor's property.

The said Licence shall be subject to the provisions and restrictions hereinafter contained.

1.2 The Licensor confirms that he is the freehold (or otherwise entitled) owner of the Licensor's property and has the authority to grant this Licence for itself or any tenants or Lessees with any right or interest in the Licensor's property.

2 Licence Fee

That in consideration of the granting of this Licence, the Licensee shall pay to the Licensor the sum of £ _____ for every week or part thereof, commencing the _____ and for the duration that the Licensee's scaffold is in place. Payment is to be made monthly in advance.

3 Termination of Licence

That this Licence shall:

(a) Subject to the provisions of Clause 11 hereof, the duration of the Licence granted by Clause 1 shall be for a term of not more than 12 months commencing not later than _____

(b) The Licensee may, by written notice to the Licensor such notice to be served no later than 30 days prior to the expiration of the 12 month period referred to in (a) above, extend the duration of this licence for a further period of up to a maximum of 12 months.

(c) On the expiration of the 12 month period referred to in (a) above, this Licence may be renewed with the Licensor's express consent at a Licence fee to be agreed between the parties (being no less than the fee payable hereunder) whereupon a renewed Licence shall commence and run from month to month determinable by either party on one month's previous notice in writing.

4 Consents and Certificates for Scaffolding

That the Licensee will obtain and maintain in force all necessary consents whether formally or otherwise in connection with the Licensee's scaffold and will, on demand, produce evidence to the Licensor's reasonable satisfaction that there are in existence up to date consents for the Licensee's scaffold.

5 The Scaffold and Equipment in Use

That in erecting, using and striking the scaffolding the following standards are to be applied:

(a) Prior to the erection of the scaffold and throughout the time that it is in situ at the Licensor's property and upon its dismantling to observe and comply with all statutory regulations, and by-laws in relation thereto.

(b) No nuisance, damage or annoyance shall be occasioned to the Licensor, his Lessees, Tenants and invitees during the erection, operation and maintenance and dismantling of the scaffold and only properly skilled persons shall undertake these tasks.

(c) To ensure that proper precautions are taken (in addition to complying with all statutory requirements) in the transport, construction, erection, maintenance, operation and dismantling of the scaffold.

6 Indemnity

That the Licensee either directly or through the provision of a contract for the works is to indemnify the Licensor from and against all reasonable actions, costs, losses, or liabilities whatsoever and howsoever arising out of or in connection with or by reason of the Licensee's scaffold and shall insure or cause to be insured such risks to the reasonable satisfaction of the Licensor with a minimum limit to indemnity of £2,000,000 and on demand shall produce to the Licensor the policy or policies of such further evidence as becomes necessary for the duration of the Licence and a note of the Licensor's interest shall be endorsed on the Schedule to the Policy.

7 Rectification of any Damage Caused by the Use of the Scaffold and Equipment

In the event of any damage or injury of any kind whatsoever being caused to the Licensor's property or any of its contents in any manner arising from the exercise of this Licence, the Licensee shall, if so required by the Licensor (and if so required by the Licensor with the Contractors chosen by the Licensor) immediately commence the making good, repair or rectification of such damage or injury and to proceed diligently and expeditiously therewith and such making good, repair or rectification shall be to the reasonable satisfaction of the Licensor. In default thereof, the Licensor may undertake or procure the undertaking of the making good, repair or rectification and the Licensee shall pay the cost of carrying out the same on demand.

8 No Relationship of Landlord and Tenant

That neither this Licence nor anything done by the Licensor in pursuance thereof or in relation thereto shall be deemed to create between the Licensor and the Licensee, the relationship of Landlord and Tenant and the law and enactment relating to Landlord and Tenant shall not apply to this Licence. In furtherance of the intention expressed above and for the avoidance of doubt, it is hereby specifically confirmed and acknowledged by the Licensee that at no time throughout the duration of this Licence will the Licensee enjoy the right to exclusive physical possession of land and of the air space as against the Licensor.

9 Interpretation

That for the purpose of this Licence it is agreed as follows:

(a) Reference in the Licence to the Licensor and the Licensee shall, where the context so admits, be deemed to include a reference to their respective successors in Title and assigns and all persons duly authorised by them.

(b) The clause headings shall not affect the interpretation of the Licence.

(c) Any Notice served under or in connection with this Licence shall be properly served if it complies with the provisions of Section 196 of the Law of Property Act 1925 (as amended by the Recorded Delivery Service Act 1962).

(d) Any reference in this Licence to any provision of statute shall be construed as a reference to that provision as replaced, amended or re-enacted at the relevant time and shall include any subordinate legislation or regulation made under any of the foregoing.

10 Costs

That the Licensee will immediately, on signing hereof, pay the proper Surveyor's fees, costs and disbursement plus VAT incurred by the Licensor of and incidental to the preparation and completion of this Licence in the sum of £ _____ plus VAT and that in the event of any damage or disturbance being occasioned to the Licensor's property and the rectification of the same as provided for in Clause 7 hereof, the Licensee shall defray the proper legal, Surveyors' and, if appropriate, Structural Engineers' costs plus disbursements and VAT immediately upon the production to the Licensee of appropriate invoices in respect of such fees arising from any incident of damage.

11 That the Licensor and the Licensee further agree:

(a) In the event of the Licensee being in breach of any of its agreements under the terms thereof and shall have failed to remedy such breach (if the same is remediable) as soon as reasonably practicable but in any event within fourteen days of receipt of such a request by the licensor to remedy such breach this Licence may be terminated.

(b) In the event of this Licence being terminated for whatever reason then such termination shall be without prejudice to any rights of action or remedies which may have accrued to the licensor in respect of the terms hereof.

In Witness whereof we have set our hands

this _____ day of _____ (month) _____ (year)

*Signed for and on behalf of _____

_____ *Duly Authorised Agent

Licensor _____

* Witness to the signature of Licensor (authorised signatory)

Name _____

Address _____

Occupation _____

*Signed for and on behalf of

_____ *Duly Authorised Agent

Licensee _____

* Witness to the signature of Licensee (authorised signatory)

Name _____

Address _____

Occupation _____

*Delete as necessary

This Licence has been prepared by

_____

(Insert name and address of Architect's practice)

Licence   **Waive certain rights**

An Agreement by way of Licence

to waive certain rights to air space

during the development of

_____

(Insert here address of site)

and air space during the development of

_____

(Insert here address of site)

development site

Whereas

in this Licence the following expressions are to have the meanings described therein:

"The Licensor"	shall mean

_____

(Insert here name of the owner of the adjoining property)

"The Licensor's Property"	shall mean the land and premises thereon known as

_____

(Insert here address of property above which the jib will oversail)

"The Licensee"	shall mean

_____

(Insert here name of developer or his contractor, as appropriate)

"The Licensee's Property"	shall mean the land comprising the site known as

_____

(Insert here address of development site)

development site shown for the purposes of identification only edged green on the plan annexed hereto ("the Plan")

"The Licensee's Crane"	shall mean the crane to be used by the Licensee, the lifting jib of which will, from time to time, pass through the air space above the Licensor's property to the extent detailed on the plan annexed hereto ("the Plan")

And Whereas

the Licensee intends to carry out work to the Licensee's property but will require the use of a tower crane (hereinafter called the Licensee's crane) to facilitate the prompt completion of the said works

And Whereas

the Licensor hereby confirms that the right to the air above the Licensor's property is vested in their title to the said property

Now the Licensor and the Licensee
do hereby agree
to enter into this licence as follows

1 Granting of Licence

That in consideration of the undertakings and conditions hereinafter reserved and contained, the Licensor hereby grants to the Licensee by way of Licence permission to transport, erect, install, repair, maintain, operate and dismantle with all necessary and usual ancillary works the Licensee's crane on the Licensee's property notwithstanding that the lifting jibs of the Licensee's crane, the approximate position and radius of which is identified on the plan (and no other part or parts of the Licensee's crane whatsoever) shall, at various times, oversail the Licensor's property but at no time shall any loads oversail the Licensor's property provided always that the said Licence shall be subject to the provisions and restrictions hereinafter contained.

2 Licence Fee

That in consideration of the granting of this Licence, the Licensee shall pay to the Licensor the sum of £ _____ for every week or part thereof, commencing the _____ and for the duration that the Licensee's crane is in place. Payment is to be made monthly in advance.

3 Termination of Licence

That this Licence shall:

(a) Subject to the provisions of Clause 11 hereof, the duration of the Licence granted by Clause 1 shall be for a term of not more than 12 months commencing not later than _____

(b) On the expiration of the 12 month period referred to in (a) above, this Licence may be renewed with the Licensor's express consent at a Licence fee to be agreed between the parties (being no less than the fee payable hereunder) whereupon a renewed Licence shall commence and run from month to month determinable by either party on one month's previous notice in writing.

4 Consents and Test Certificate for Crane

That the Licensee will obtain and maintain in force all necessary consents whether formally or otherwise in connection with the Licensee's crane and will, on demand, produce evidence to the Licensor's reasonable satisfaction that there is in existence an up to date Test Certificate for the Licensee's crane.

5 The Crane in Use

That in erecting, using and striking the crane the following standards are to be applied:

(a) Prior to the erection of the crane and throughout the time that it is in situ at the Licensor's property and upon its dismantling to observe and comply with all statutory regulations, regulations and by-laws in relation thereto.

(b) No nuisance, damage or annoyance (including but not limited to interference with any radio, television or other transmission signals) shall be occasioned to the Licensor, his Lessees, Tenants and invitees during the erection, operation and maintenance and dismantling of the crane and only properly skilled persons shall undertake these tasks.

(c) To ensure that proper precautions are taken (in addition to complying with all statutory requirements) in the transport, construction, erection, maintenance, operation and dismantling of the crane.

6 Indemnity	That the Licensee either directly or through the provision of a contract for the works is to indemnify the Licensor from and against all reasonable actions, costs, losses, or liabilities whatsoever and howsoever arising out of or in connection with or by reason of the Licensee's crane and shall insure or cause to be insured such risks to the reasonable satisfaction of the Licensor with a minimum limit to indemnity of £ _____ and on demand shall produce to the Licensor the policy or policies or such further evidence as becomes necessary for the duration of the licence and a note of the Licensor's interest shall be endorsed on the Schedule to the Policy.
7 Rectification of Any Damage Caused by the Use of the Crane	In the event of any damage or injury of any kind whatsoever being caused to the Licensor' property or any of its contents in any manner arising from the exercise of this Licence, the Licensee shall, if so required by the Licensor (and if so required by the Licensor with the Contractors chosen by the Licensor) immediately commence the making good, repair or rectification of such damage or injury and to proceed diligently and expeditiously therewith and such making good, repair or rectification shall be to the reasonable satisfaction of the Licensor. In default thereof, the Licensor may undertake or procure the undertaking of the making good, repair or rectification and the Licensee shall pay the cost of carrying out the same on demand.
8 No Relationship of Landlord and Tenant	That neither this Licence nor anything done by the Licensor in pursuance thereof or in relation thereto shall be deemed to create between the Licensor and the Licensee, the relationship of Landlord and Tenant and the law and enactment relating to Landlord and Tenant shall not apply to this Licence. In furtherance of the intention expressed above and for the avoidance of doubt, it is hereby specifically confirmed and acknowledged by the Licensee that at no time throughout the duration of this Licence will the Licensee enjoy the right to exclusive physical possession of the air space as against the Licensor.
9 Interpretation	That for the purpose of this Licence it is agreed as follows: (a) Reference in the Licence to the Licensor and the Licensee shall, where the context so admits, be deemed to include a reference to their respective successors in title and assigns and all persons duly authorised by them. (b) The clause headings shall not affect the interpretation of the licence. (c) Any Notice served under or in connection with this Licence shall be properly served if it complies with the provisions of Section 196 of the Law of Property Act 1925 (as amended by the Recorded Delivery Service Act 1962). (d) Any reference in this Licence to any provision of statute shall be construed as a reference to that provision as replaced, amended or re-enacted at the relevant time and shall include any subordinate legislation or regulation made under any of the foregoing.
10 Costs	That the Licensee will immediately, on signing hereof, pay the proper Surveyors' fees, costs and disbursement plus VAT incurred by the Licensor of and incidental to the preparation and completion of this Licence in the sum of £ _____ plus VAT and that in the event of any damage or disturbance being occasioned to the Licensor's property and the rectification of the same as provided for in Clause 7 hereof, the Licensee shall defray the proper legal, Surveyors' and, if appropriate, Structural Engineers' costs plus disbursements and VAT immediately upon the production to the Licensee of appropriate invoices in respect of such fees arising from any incident of damage.

11 That the Licensor and the Licensee further agree:

(a) In the event of the Licensee being in breach of any of its agreements under the terms thereof and shall have failed to remedy such breach (if the same is remediable) as soon as reasonably practicable but in any event within fourteen days of receipt of such a request by the Licensor to remedy such breach this Licence may be terminated forthwith.

(b) In the event of this Licence being terminated for whatever reason then such termination shall be without prejudice to any rights of action or remedies which may have accrued to the Licensor in respect of the terms hereof.

In Witness whereof we have set our hands

this _____ day of _____ (month) _____ (year)

*Signed for and on behalf of _____

_____ *Duly Authorised Agent*

Licensor _____

* Witness to the signature of Licensor (authorised signatory)

Name _____

Address _____

Occupation _____

*Signed for and on behalf of

_____ *Duly Authorised Agent*

Licensee _____

* Witness to the signature of Licensee (authorised signatory)

Name _____

Address _____

Occupation _____

Delete as necessary

Index

Index